MATHEMATICS FOR NURSING SCIENCE
A PROGRAMMED TEXT

SALLY IRENE LIPSEY
Brooklyn College
of the
City University of New York

Second Edition

A Wiley Medical Publication
JOHN WILEY & SONS
New York / London / Sydney / Toronto

Library of Congress Cataloging in Publication Data:

Lipsey, Sally Irene.
    Mathematics for nursing science.

    (A Wiley medical publication)
    Includes index.
    1. Nursing—Mathematics—Programmed instruction.
I. Title.
RT68.L56 1976   513'.02'4613   76-44843
ISBN 0-471-01798-1 (pbk)

Printed in the United States of America

10 9 8 7 6 5 4 3 2 1

MATHEMATICS FOR NURSING SCIENCE

To Marion, Carol, and Eleanor

PREFACE

I am happy, of course, that so many people have found my book useful. The purpose of the text was and remains the achievement of thorough understanding of fundamental principles. Mechanical methods are eschewed because they often become jumbled in students' minds. To provide more opportunity for practice with these fundamental principles, the second edition contains new material on applications to dosage problems, including concrete examples from nursing situations involving oral and parenteral administration. The section on measurements has additional material on converting from one system to another. We also provided eight new sets of drill exercises. The last section of this edition contains a discussion of the pocket calculator with illustrative problems. It shows how to make use of this helpful device while demonstrating that it is impossible to use it without clear understanding of the principles emphasized throughout the book.

The text is designed to serve well-prepared students as well as those who need extra practice. There are whole sections, drill frames called "subframes," and pages of extra exercises which students may work on or skip over, according to their results on the numerous self-testing instruments. Instructors may select for assignment the portions of the text most suitable for the type of course being given.

The first edition was devoted mainly to teaching. The second edition retains this feature but also may now be used as a handy reference. We have expanded the Contents, added an index, and provided a portable card of Tables of Equivalents. Summaries after each section highlight, illustrate, and review principles taught in the programmed explanations.

I am most grateful to those who have made suggestions for the text, especially Allene Pearson, R.N., of Del Mar College, Corpus Christi, Texas, Shirley R. Burke, R.N., of the Community College of Allegheny County, and Joyce Le Fever Kee of the University of Delaware. Carl Q. Keller, Medical Operations Manager of Pfizer, Inc., and Sidney Rubinstein, pharmacist, very kindly provided me with a variety of the latest pharmaceutical literature. I appreciate very much the assistance I received from Eleanor Lipsey and Marion Lipsey in typing and checking the manuscript. To my colleagues at John Wiley, Inc., especially Earl Shepherd, many thanks for all your excellent help.

September 1976   S. I. L.

PREFACE TO FIRST EDITION

Among all the important tasks that a nurse may be called upon to perform, one of the most significant to the safety and welfare of the patient, is that of administering drugs and observing and recording their effects. The capable nurse reads and understands prescriptions, carries out doctors' orders, records what he or she has done and how the patient has reacted. All of these activities require the use of some aspect of elementary mathematics.

In his or her encounter with prescriptions and orders, a nurse must be able to deal with either of the systems of weights and measures which are in common use in the United States today: the apothecaries' system and the metric system. He or she must also be able to convert measurements from one system to the other. Even where the most modern facilities and services are available, the nurse may find it necessary to calculate the amount of drug required to make a given solution of stated strength, to prepare a dilute solution from a more concentrated stock solution, or to prepare fractional doses from tablets. Sometimes only household measuring devices are at hand, and approximations must be made as reasonably as possible. It is clear that if the nurse does not calculate accurately, the result may be harmful to the patient.

The purpose of this book, then, is to help nursing students, working by themselves, to review the basic mathematics needed for courses in nursing science, pharmacology, and chemistry. The topics covered have been found important for both the study and the practice of nursing. These include the fundamental arithmetic operations applied to decimal and common fractions, ratio, proportion, and percentage.

We call this book a programmed text. It differs from a conventional text in that the process of learning is organized into small steps that permit each student to progress at the rate suitable for him or her individually. The student finds out at each step whether he or she fully understands the material, and, if not, is given supplementary explanation and further chances to try the same type of problem again. The student need not spend time on topics he or she knows well. Where knowledge is weak, however, we hope that this new approach will help to instill the principles more firmly.

The only prerequisite for taking this program is ability to add, subtract, multiply, and divide whole numbers.

The writing of this program was inspired by discussions with several leading figures in nursing education who pointed out the many mathematical difficulties that have appeared in the work of nursing students in classroom and hospital.

My introduction to nursing science educators and experts in programmed instruction was arranged by President Morris Meister and Dr. Alexander Joseph, Bronx Community College of the City University of New York, who also encouraged my experimental work at Bronx Community College.

Dr. Robert Kinsinger, New York State Department of Education, and Dr. Lassar Gotkin, Institute for Developmental Studies, first suggested the need for this text and supplied advice and encouragement as the work progressed.

I received many helpful comments and suggestions from nursing faculty, particularly from Gerald Griffin, of the National League for Nursing, Joanne Griffin of Bronx Community College, Ruth Matheney of Nassau Community College, Barbara McCarragher of Rockland Community College, Mary Millar of the Cornell University School of Nursing, Mildred Montag of Teachers College, Columbia University, and Carolyn Schwab of Brooklyn College.

I am grateful to Erwin Just, Chairman of the Department of Mathematics at Bronx Community College, and to Edith Nielsen and Dorothy White, Chairman of the Nursing Science Department of Brooklyn College and Rockland Community College, respectively, for useful discussions of testing procedure and for permission to try out the text at their institutions.

I benefited greatly from the guidance of members of the faculty of Teachers College, Columbia University, especially Howard Fehr, Myron Rosskopf, and Phil Lange.

I am indebted to Dr. Robert Lipsey for a critical reading of the text. Thanks are also due to Flora Rothstein, and Ann and Meyer Lipsey without whose help this book could never have been written.

S. I. L.

CONTENTS

MATHEMATICS FOR
NURSING SCIENCE

COMMON FRACTIONS
INTRODUCTION

Tablets come in certain stock sizes. For instance, a tablet may contain 8 milligrams of morphine sulfate. If a patient is required to have 2 milligrams, the nurse must be able to calculate what part of the tablet to use. If a vial of medicine had contained $7\frac{1}{4}$ ounces, and $2\frac{3}{4}$ ounces had been used, would you be able to calculate how much was on hand? Suppose 48 tablets containing atropine sulfate gr. $\frac{1}{50}$ were left in the supply cabinet for administration in dosages of gr. $\frac{1}{150}$. Would you be able to calculate how many doses could be administered? Drugs are sometimes available in a limited number of stock solutions; the nurse may need to alter the stock solutions for a given patient's requirements and thus find that knowledge of fractions is essential.

In this and succeeding sections we discuss common fractions. Section 6 is devoted to decimal fractions. Here we review enough about common fractions so the student is able to:

1. Solve simple verbal problems requiring the formation of a common fraction.

2. Use the appropriate vocabulary for the terms of a fraction.

3. Judge the relative sizes of quantities represented by fractions.

4. Add and subtract fractions with like denominators.

5. Convert from one form of numeral to another, such as from an improper fraction to a mixed number.

PROFICIENCY GAUGE

It is possible that you do not need to review the topics of Section 1. Gauge your proficiency by working out the following exercises. Then check your answers with those given below.

1. A gallon is divided into 8 pints. Each pint is what part of the gallon?

2. If 5 drams of a powdered drug are mixed with 2 drams of sugar, what part of the total mixture is the drug?

3. What is the numerator of the fraction $\frac{8}{17}$? What is the other number called?

4. Which fraction is greater, $\frac{1}{8}$ or $\frac{1}{9}$?

5. Which fraction represents the smallest quantity, $\frac{7}{10}$, $\frac{5}{12}$, or $\frac{7}{12}$?

6. Add: $\frac{20}{43} + \frac{10}{43} + \frac{11}{43}$.

7. Subtract: $\frac{7}{11} - \frac{2}{11}$.

8. Attach the adjectives "proper" or "improper" to each of the following fractions: $\frac{2}{3}, \frac{2}{7}, \frac{3}{4}, \frac{4}{3}, \frac{4}{5}, \frac{9}{7}$.

9. Change $\frac{23}{5}$ to a mixed number.

10. Circle the improper fractions in the following list and change them to mixed numbers: $\frac{19}{12}, \frac{3}{5}, \frac{99}{4}, \frac{11}{2}, \frac{8}{8}, \frac{8}{5}$.

11. Change $3\frac{7}{8}$ to an improper fraction.

. . . .

Answers

1. $\frac{1}{8}$

2. $\frac{5}{7}$

3. The numerator is 8. The denominator is 17.

4. $\frac{1}{8}$

5. $\frac{5}{12}$

6. $\frac{41}{43}$

7. $\frac{5}{11}$

8. $\frac{2}{3}$, proper; $\frac{2}{7}$, proper; $\frac{3}{4}$, proper; $\frac{4}{3}$, improper; $\frac{4}{5}$, proper; $\frac{9}{7}$, improper

9. $4\frac{3}{5}$

10. $\frac{19}{12} = 1\frac{7}{12}$, $\frac{99}{4} = 24\frac{3}{4}$, $\frac{11}{2} = 5\frac{1}{2}$, $\frac{8}{8} = 1$, $\frac{8}{5} = 1\frac{3}{5}$

11. $\frac{31}{8}$

If you have no errors, read "To the Student," below, skip Section 1, and start with Section 2.

TO THE STUDENT

Each topic is organized into units of information presented in "frames." In most cases, you supply some of the information. For almost every frame, you are required to fill in your own words or symbols. Your responding helps you to learn *more than anything else.*

Each frame is followed on the left by the correct answer and on the right by an explanation. Cover the entire part of the page below the frame on which you are working. We will supply an answer shield. After you have completed your response to the frame, uncover the answer and discussion. If your response is correct (in your own words, of course), you can proceed with confidence. You need not read the discussion. If your response is incorrect, use the explanation to correct your work. If you correct your work carefully, you will solve the next problem perfectly.

For many frames, there are subframes that give you a chance to try the same type of problem over again. Ignore these subframes wherever you know the work so well that you do not need the extra practice.

You may notice that fractions appear in two different forms for convenience in printing. Some are made with a slanted line ($\frac{1}{2}$). Others have a horizontal bar ($\frac{1}{2}$). The meaning is the same in both cases.

Meaning of a Fraction

A fraction (or simple ratio) is a symbol representing one or more of the equal parts into which a whole quantity or several whole quantities have been subdivided.

---

1. Picture yourself dividing the entire contents of a bottle of medicine into 8 equal portions. Each portion would be what fractional part of the whole supply?

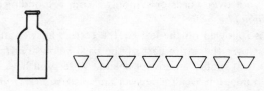

. . . .

$\bigtriangledown = \dfrac{1}{8}$

---

2. When you cut a pie into 4 equal parts, each piece is what part of the whole pie?

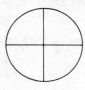

. . . .

$\dfrac{1}{4}$

---

3. Your last answer, ¼, represents 1 of the 4 parts into which the whole pie was subdivided. Three of 4 parts into which the pie was subdivided would be represented by _____ .

. . . .

$\dfrac{3}{4}$

---

4. A typical dose of magnesium carbonate as an antacid is 600 milligrams (mg.). Each 100 milligrams is what part of the typical dose? If a patient is given only 200 mg., what part of a typical dose has he been given?

. . . .

$\frac{1}{6}$; $\frac{2}{6}$ or $\frac{1}{3}$

5. If a student correctly answers 115 out of 137 questions on an achievement test, write his score as a fraction. In other words, what fraction represents the part of the test that was done correctly?

. . . .

$\frac{115}{137}$ $score = \dfrac{number\ of\ correct\ answers}{number\ of\ answers} = \dfrac{115}{137}$

6. Suppose you have mixed 2 ounces of sugar with 3 ounces of flour. How many ounces of the combination would you have? What part of the *total* mixture is *sugar*?

. . . .

5; $\frac{2}{5}$ $\dfrac{number\ of\ ounces\ of\ sugar}{number\ of\ ounces\ of\ total\ mixture} = \dfrac{2}{5}$

6a.

A class consists of 17 men and 19 women. What is the ratio of men to the total number of students (i.e., what fractional part of the total is male)?

. . . .

$\frac{17}{36}$ $\dfrac{number\ of\ men}{total\ number\ in\ class} = \dfrac{17}{17+19} = \dfrac{17}{36}$

Terms of a Fraction

Think of any fraction or ratio, ½, ¾, ⅞, etc. The number above the line (1, 3, 7, etc.) is called the numerator; the number underneath the line (2, 4, 8, etc.) is called the denominator. A way to distinguish between them is to remember that the <u>d</u>enominator is <u>d</u>own below the line, and represents the number of parts into which a given whole object or quantity has been broken or subdivided. The numerator is <u>up</u> above the line and represents the number of parts selected.

---

7. In which of the following fractions are the denominators greater than 5?

$$\frac{2}{3}, \frac{5}{12}, \frac{4}{7}, \frac{11}{20}, \frac{7}{3}$$

. . . .

$$\frac{5}{12}, \frac{4}{7}, \frac{11}{20}$$

12, 7 and 20 are the denominators greater than 5.

---

8. The (denominator/numerator) of the fraction ⅖ is 2.

. . . .

numerator

8a.

The (denominator/numerator) of the ratio ¾ is 4.

. . . .

denominator

---

9. Until the 16th century, fractions were often called "broken numbers." They may be thought of as symbols representing one or more of the equal parts into which a whole object or quantity is "broken." What does ⅚ then represent? Which is the denominator? Which the numerator?

. . . .

⅚ may be thought of as a symbol representing 5 of 6 parts into which a quantity or set has been broken. The denominator denotes the total number of parts, 6, and the numerator represents the number of parts selected, 5.

---

10. What does ⅘ represent? Which is larger—the numerator or the denominator?

. . . .

⅘ is a symbol representing 4 of 5 parts of a quantity. The denominator, 5, representing the total number of parts, is larger.

---

11. What does ⁵⁄₉ represent? ⁷⁄₉? Which is greater, ⁵⁄₉ or ⁷⁄₉?

. . . .

⁵⁄₉ represents 5 of 9 given parts; ⁷⁄₉ represents 7 of the same 9 parts; ⁷⁄₉ is greater than ⁵⁄₉.

---

12. You should now be able to define fraction, numerator, and denominator. Write out your definitions. Then check with page 25, Items 1 and 2.

Relative Size

The relative sizes of fractions may be judged by keeping denominators fixed and comparing numerators or by keeping numerators fixed and comparing denominators.

---

13. At a party, the hostess cut a pork sausage into 8 equal pieces for hors d'oeuvres. John ate 3 pieces and Mary ate 5 pieces. What fractional portion of the sausage did John eat? What fractional portion did Mary eat?

. . . .

John ate $\frac{3}{8}$ of the sausage; Mary ate $\frac{5}{8}$ of the sausage.

---

14. Refer to the frame above. Obviously (John/Mary) is the guest who had the bigger portion, and of the two fractions ($\frac{3}{8}$ / $\frac{5}{8}$) must represent the bigger amount.

. . . .

Mary had the bigger portion; $\frac{5}{8}$ must represent the bigger amount.

---

15. Picture Tom, Dick, and Harry cutting a very long sausage into 23 equal pieces. Tom ate $^8/_{23}$ of the sausage, Dick ate $^4/_{23}$, and Harry ate $^{11}/_{23}$. Who ate the least? the most?

. . . .

Dick, least; Harry, most

16. Of the following fractions, which has the least value? the greatest? What is the same about all of them? $\dfrac{17}{19}, \dfrac{11}{19}, \dfrac{13}{19}, \dfrac{5}{19}$

. . . .

$\dfrac{5}{19}$, least; $\dfrac{17}{19}$, most; the denominator, 19

16a.

Of the following fractions, which is least? greatest? What is the same in all? $\dfrac{1}{12}, \dfrac{11}{12}, \dfrac{7}{12}, \dfrac{5}{12}$

. . . .

$\dfrac{1}{12}$, least; $\dfrac{11}{12}$, greatest; the denominator, 12

17. Which is less, $^7/_{12}$ or $^{11}/_{12}$? State your reason.

. . . .

$\dfrac{7}{12}$ is less than $\dfrac{11}{12}$, since the denominators are equal and 11 is greater than 7.

18. Imagine a brick of ice cream being divided equally into 4 portions. Then imagine a similar brick of ice cream divided into 6 equal portions, instead. In which case would the portions be larger? Why?

. . . .

In the first case. The smaller the number of portions, the larger each portion must be. The larger the number of portions, the smaller each portion must be.

19. Which patient has the greater dose, the one receiving ⅓ grain or the one receiving ¼ grain? (Assume that the ingredients are alike.) Think back to the definition of a fraction.

. . . .

A dose of ⅓ grain means 1 of 3 parts into which the grain has been divided, and a dose of ¼ grain means 1 of 4 parts into which the grain has been divided. The more parts into which a quantity is divided, the smaller each part must be. Therefore, ⅓ is greater than ¼.

19a.

Which is greater, ¼ or ⅙? Why? (Notice that the denominators are different.)

. . . .

If a quantity is divided into 4 equal parts, each part would be ¼. If the same quantity is divided into 6 equal parts, each part would be ⅙. The smaller the number of subdivisions, the larger each part would be. Thus ¼ must be greater than ⅙.

---

20. The quantities ¾ grain and 3/7 grain have (the same numerators/different numerators). The fraction ¾ represents (fewer/more) subdivisions of the grain than the fraction 3/7. ¾ is (greater/less) than 3/7.

. . . .

the same numerators; fewer; greater than

20a.

Compare 1/12 grain with 1/10 grain. The quantity 1/12 grain represents (fewer/more) subdivisions of the grain and is (greater/less) than 1/10.

. . . .

more; less

Twelve subdivisions are more than 10. Each of 12 subdivisions of a grain is smaller than each of 10 subdivisions. Thus 1/12 is less than 1/10.

21. If two fractions have the same numerator, the fraction with the smaller denominator represents (fewer/more) subdivisions and (smaller/greater) size.

. . . .

fewer; greater

Consider $\frac{2}{3}$ and $\frac{2}{5}$. The fraction with the smaller denominator, $\frac{2}{3}$, represents 3 subdivisions of an object or set. The fraction $\frac{2}{5}$ represents 5 subdivisions. Each of the 3 subdivisions must be larger than each of the 5 subdivisions.

21a.

If two fractions have the same numerator, the fraction with the larger denominator represents (fewer/more) subdivisions and (smaller/greater) size.

. . . .

more; smaller

The more subdivisions there are, the smaller each subdivision must be.

22. Think of any two different fractions with the *same numerator*. The greater the denominator, the (greater/smaller) the fraction.

. . . .

smaller

22a.

Think of any two fractions with the *same numerator*. The smaller the denominator, the (greater/smaller) the fraction.

. . . .

greater

23. If the numerators of two fractions are the same, the greater fraction has the (greater/smaller) denominator.

. . . .

smaller

23a.

If the numerators of two fractions are the same, the (greater/smaller) fraction has the greater denominator.

. . . .

smaller

---

24. Give an example of a fraction that is greater than $\frac{1}{4}$ and has the same denominator.

. . . .

$\frac{2}{4}, \frac{3}{4}$

---

25. A dosage of $\frac{1}{5}$ grain of drug A is too great for a certain patient. Give an example of a smaller dosage that the doctor might consider.

. . . .

Increase the denominator and decrease the fraction: $\frac{1}{6}, \frac{1}{7}, \frac{1}{8}$, etc.

25a.

A dosage of $\frac{1}{12}$ grain of drug B must be increased. Give an example of a larger dosage by changing the denominator. Give an example of a larger dosage by changing the numerator.

. . . .

$\frac{1}{11}, \frac{1}{10}, \frac{1}{9}$, etc.; $\frac{2}{12}, \frac{3}{12}, \frac{4}{12}, \frac{5}{12}$, etc. (all larger doses)

26. Suppose the numerators of two fractions are equal and the denominators are not equal. How do you know which one is greater?

. . . .

The fraction with the smaller denominator is greater.

26a.

Suppose the denominator of two fractions are equal and the numerators are not equal. How do you know which one is greater?

. . . .

The fraction with the larger numerator is greater.

27. For the following pairs of fractions, circle the greater fraction:

(a) $\frac{2}{9}, \frac{5}{9}$ (b) $\frac{3}{7}, \frac{3}{4}$ (c) $\frac{1}{5}, \frac{1}{6}$ (d) $\frac{5}{7}, \frac{3}{7}$

. . . .

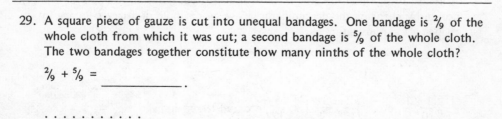

(a) $\left(\frac{5}{9}\right)$;   (b) $\left(\frac{3}{4}\right)$;   (c) $\left(\frac{1}{5}\right)$;   (d) $\left(\frac{5}{7}\right)$

28. You should now be able to state the principle to be followed in comparing the sizes of fractions. Assume that two given fractions have equal numerators, and state the principle to be followed in selecting the greater. Then assume that two given fractions have equal denominators and state the principle to be followed in selecting the greater. Check with page 25, Item 3.

Addition or Subtraction of Fractions With Like Denominators
Add or subtract the numerators and keep the denominator.

29. A square piece of gauze is cut into unequal bandages. One bandage is $\frac{2}{9}$ of the whole cloth from which it was cut; a second bandage is $\frac{5}{9}$ of the whole cloth. The two bandages together constitute how many ninths of the whole cloth?

$\frac{2}{9} + \frac{5}{9} =$ _____ .

. . . .

7 ninths; $\frac{7}{9}$

29a.

Given two doses of atropine, $^3/_{100}$ grain and $^{15}/_{100}$ grain, the total dosage would be _____ grain.

. . . .

$\dfrac{18}{100}$

$$\dfrac{3}{100} + \dfrac{15}{100} = \dfrac{3 + 15}{100} = \dfrac{18}{100}$$

$\dfrac{18}{100}$ *may be reduced to* $\dfrac{9}{50}$

30. The sum of fractions with the same denominator may be found by_____ _____ . Solve the following problem or problems that illustrate this statement:

(a) $\dfrac{5}{9} + \dfrac{3}{9} =$ _____   (b) $\dfrac{2}{7} + \dfrac{2}{9} =$ _____

, , , , , , , , , , , , ,

adding the numerators; (a) $\dfrac{8}{9}$; (b) The sum must be found by first changing both fractions to equivalent fractions with the same denominator, as you will see in Section 2.

30a.

Add the following ratios: $\dfrac{4}{11} + \dfrac{6}{11} =$ _____ .

. . . .

$\dfrac{10}{11}$

31. $\dfrac{2}{21} + \dfrac{17}{21} =$ _____ .

. . . .

$\dfrac{19}{21}$

31a.

$$\frac{19}{50} + \frac{3}{50} = \underline{\hspace{3cm}}.$$

. . . .

$$\frac{22}{50} \text{ or } \frac{11}{25}$$

32. Subtract: $\frac{7}{9} - \frac{2}{9} = \underline{\hspace{3cm}}.$

. . . .

$$\frac{5}{9}$$

32a.

$$\frac{11}{20} - \frac{2}{20} = \underline{\hspace{3cm}}.$$

. . . .

$$\frac{9}{20}$$

33. The difference of fractions with the same denominator may be found by
_____. Solve the following problem or
problems that illustrate this statement:

(a) $\frac{3}{4} - \frac{1}{4} = \underline{\hspace{2cm}}$ (b) $\frac{7}{9} - \frac{2}{9} = \underline{\hspace{2cm}}$

(c) $\frac{9}{7} - \frac{9}{2} = \underline{\hspace{2cm}}$

. . . .

subtracting the numerators; (a) $\frac{2}{4}$ or $\frac{1}{2}$; (b) $\frac{5}{9}$

33a.

Subtract the following ratios: $\dfrac{10}{11} - \dfrac{4}{11} =$ _____.

. . . .

$\dfrac{6}{11}$

33b.

Subtract the following ratios: $\dfrac{10}{100} - \dfrac{3}{100} =$ _____.

. . . .

$\dfrac{7}{100}$

---

34. You should now be able to state a principle for adding or subtracting fractions with the same denominators. Check with p. 25, Item 4.

Unity Expressed as a Fraction

Each fraction with a numerator equal to its denominator has the value 1. This enables us to simplify results.

---

35. To consolidate the supply of a nonsterile antiseptic solution, the contents of one bottle containing $\frac{3}{8}$ quart are combined with the contents of another containing $\frac{5}{8}$ quart. The combined contents (will/will not) fit into a 1 quart bottle.

. . . .

will

$\frac{3}{8} + \frac{5}{8} = \frac{8}{8}$. *The contents will fit into a 1=quart bottle since $\frac{8}{8}$ represents all 8 of the 8 parts into which 1 quart may be divided. Symbolically, then, $\frac{8}{8} = 1$.*

35a.

Given 1 grain, into how many fifths may the whole be divided? $(1 = \dfrac{?}{5})$ Into how many sevenths? $(1 = \dfrac{?}{7})$ Into how many twentieths? $(1 = \dfrac{?}{20})$

. . . .

One grain may be divided into 5 equal parts $(1 = \frac{5}{5})$ or 7 equal parts $(1 = \frac{7}{7})$ or 20 equal parts $(1 = \frac{20}{20})$ or n equal parts $(1 = \frac{n}{n})$.

---

36. Express 1 as a fraction with the denominator 3. (Into how many thirds may a whole be divided?)

. . . .

$1 = \frac{3}{3}$ (The whole may be divided into 3 thirds.)

---

37. Simplify $\frac{16}{16}$.

. . . .

$$\frac{16}{16} = 1$$

---

38. If 1 is expressed as a fraction, the numerator is (greater than/equal to/less than) the denominator, for every possible denominator.

. . . .

If 1 is expressed as a fraction, the numerator *is equal to the denominator*.

$1 = \frac{2}{2} = \frac{3}{3} = \frac{4}{4} = \frac{5}{5} = \ldots = \frac{n}{n}$, etc. See p. 25, Item 5.

Types of Fractions

Number symbols may be classified into proper and improper fractions, mixed numbers, and whole numbers. In order to carry out arithmetical operations, it is important to know how to convert from one type of symbol to another.

---

39. Definition: A proper fraction is a fraction with a numerator less than the denominator, for example, $\frac{1}{2}, \frac{1}{3}, \frac{2}{3}, \frac{1}{4}, \frac{2}{4}, \frac{3}{4}, \frac{1}{5}, \frac{17}{39}, \frac{210}{529}$. Give an example of a proper fraction having a denominator of 7.

. . . .

The following are all proper fractions having a denominator of 7: $\frac{1}{7}, \frac{2}{7}, \frac{3}{7}, \frac{4}{7}, \frac{5}{7}, \frac{6}{7}$.

---

40. Circle all the proper fractions in the following set: $\dfrac{1}{5}, \dfrac{2}{7}, \dfrac{3}{2}, \dfrac{5}{9}, \dfrac{17}{25}, \dfrac{25}{17}, \dfrac{7}{3}, \dfrac{9}{9}$.

. . . .

$\left(\dfrac{1}{5}\right), \left(\dfrac{2}{7}\right), \left(\dfrac{5}{9}\right), \left(\dfrac{17}{25}\right)$ *These are the only fractions in which the numerator is less than the denominator.*

40a.

Circle all the proper fractions in the following set: $\dfrac{3}{8}, \dfrac{2}{9}, \dfrac{6}{10}, \dfrac{4}{3}, \dfrac{26}{18}, \dfrac{18}{18}, \dfrac{18}{26}, \dfrac{8}{4}$.

. . . .

$\left(\dfrac{3}{8}\right), \left(\dfrac{2}{9}\right), \left(\dfrac{6}{10}\right), \left(\dfrac{18}{26}\right)$

41. The fraction $^{15}\!/_2$ is (a proper/an improper) fraction because the numerator is not _____ the denominator.

. . . .

an improper fraction; less than

41a.

The fraction $^3\!/_3$ is (a proper/an improper) fraction because _____ _____ .

. . . .

improper; the numerator is not less than the denominator.

42. Give an example of an improper fraction having a denominator of 12.

. . . .

$^{12}\!/_{12}$, $^{13}\!/_{12}$, $^{29}\!/_{12}$, or any fraction in which the numerator is greater than or equal to 12.

42a.

Give an example of an improper fraction having a denominator of 4.

. . . .

$\frac{4}{4}$, $\frac{5}{4}$, $\frac{6}{4}$, $\frac{7}{4}$, $\frac{8}{4}$, and so on

---

43. Next to each of the following proper fractions, write P; next to each improper fraction write I: $\frac{5}{7}$, $\frac{5}{3}$, $\frac{2}{9}$, $\frac{12}{15}$, $\frac{13}{100}$, $\frac{75}{23}$, $\frac{17}{17}$.

. . . .

P, I, P, P, P, I, I

43a.

Next to each of the following proper fractions, write P; next to each improper fraction, write I: $\frac{7}{5}$, $\frac{7}{7}$, $\frac{3}{5}$, $\frac{23}{75}$, $\frac{9}{2}$, $\frac{100}{13}$, $\frac{15}{12}$.

. . . .

I, I, P, P, I, I, I

---

44. What is a proper fraction?

. . . .

A proper fraction is a fraction in which the numerator is less than the denominator.

---

45. The value of a proper fraction is (always/sometimes/never) less than 1.

. . . .

always

In a proper fraction, the numerator is less than the denominator. If the numerator were equal to the denominator, the fraction would be equal to 1. For example, $\frac{12}{29}$ is less than $\frac{29}{29}$, which equals 1, and $\frac{7}{8}$ is less than $\frac{8}{8}$, which equals 1. Whenever the numerator is less than the denominator, the fraction must be less than 1.

---

46. Give at least three examples of an improper fraction in which the numerator is equal to the denominator.

. . . .

$\frac{1}{1}$, $\frac{2}{2}$, $\frac{3}{3}$, $\frac{4}{4}$, $\frac{5}{5}$, etc.

---

47. What is the value of any improper fraction in which the numerator is equal to the denominator?

. . . .

1

$$\frac{1}{1} = \frac{2}{2} = \frac{3}{3} = \frac{4}{4} = \frac{5}{5} = \frac{6}{6} = 1$$

---

48. Changing some improper fractions to whole numbers, we obtain the following: $\frac{1}{1} = \frac{2}{2} = \frac{3}{3} = 1; \frac{2}{1} = \frac{4}{2} = \frac{8}{4} = 2$. Complete the following: $\frac{3}{1} = \frac{6}{2} = \frac{?}{3} =$ _____. $\frac{48}{12}$ = what whole number?

. . . .

$\frac{3}{1} = \frac{6}{2} = \frac{9}{3} = 3; \frac{48}{12} = 4$

---

49. In the following list, find any improper fractions that may by changed to whole numbers, and write the whole numbers: $\frac{2}{3}, \frac{37}{12}, \frac{16}{8}, \frac{16}{16}, \frac{29}{5}, \frac{5}{29}, \frac{5}{25}, \frac{25}{5}, 1\frac{5}{8}$.

. . . .

$\dfrac{16}{8} = 2; \quad \dfrac{16}{16} = 1; \quad \dfrac{25}{5} = 5$

49a.

In the following list, circle the improper fractions that are *not* equivalent to whole numbers: $17, \dfrac{2}{3}, \dfrac{3}{2}, \dfrac{6}{5}, \dfrac{6}{6}, \dfrac{5}{6}, \dfrac{36}{12}, \dfrac{37}{12}, \dfrac{80}{40}, \dfrac{89}{40}, \dfrac{40}{89}, 2\dfrac{5}{6}.$

. . . .

$\left(\dfrac{3}{2}\right), \left(\dfrac{6}{5}\right), \left(\dfrac{37}{12}\right), \left(\dfrac{89}{40}\right)$

---

50. If a patient is given 2 tablets of identical size and swallows the whole first tablet and $\frac{1}{4}$ of the second tablet, he has swallowed $1 + \frac{1}{4}$ tablets, written $1\frac{1}{4}$. The quantity $1\frac{1}{4}$ is called a (mixed number/proper fraction).

. . . .

mixed number (the sum of a whole number and a proper fraction)

$1\frac{1}{4} = \dfrac{4}{4} + \dfrac{1}{4} = \dfrac{5}{4}$

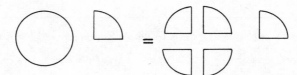

---

51. Changing an improper fraction to a mixed number, we obtain the following: $\dfrac{6}{5} = \dfrac{5}{5} + \dfrac{1}{5} = 1 + \dfrac{1}{5} = 1\frac{1}{5}$. Complete the following: $\dfrac{37}{12} = \dfrac{36}{12} + \dfrac{?}{12} = 3 + \underline{\hspace{1cm}}$

$= \underline{\hspace{2cm}}$; $\dfrac{89}{40} =$ what mixed number?

. . . .

$\dfrac{37}{12} = \dfrac{36}{12} + \dfrac{1}{12} = 3\frac{1}{12}$; $\dfrac{89}{40} = \dfrac{80}{40} + \dfrac{9}{40} = 2\frac{9}{40}$

52. Change the following fractions to mixed numbers: $\dfrac{13}{12}, \dfrac{29}{12}, \dfrac{13}{5}$.

. . . .

$1\frac{1}{12}, 2\frac{5}{12}, 2\frac{3}{5}$

---

53. What is a mixed number?

. . . .

A mixed number is the sum of a whole number and a proper fraction.

---

54. Next to each number in the following list write P if it is a proper fraction, I if it is an improper fraction, W if it is a whole number, and M if it is a mixed number: $2\frac{9}{10}, \frac{13}{5}, \frac{11}{19}, 11\frac{23}{35}, \frac{1}{2}, \frac{2}{1}, \frac{2}{3}, \frac{1}{3}, 1\frac{1}{3}, \frac{3}{1}, 3, 3\frac{1}{3}$.

. . . .

M, I, P, M, P, I, I, P, M, I, W, M

54a.

Using the same instructions as in Frame 54, label the following list: $3\frac{10}{11}, 4\frac{2}{5}$, $\frac{14}{6}, 4, \frac{12}{23}, \frac{5}{1}, 12\frac{24}{37}, 2\frac{1}{4}, \frac{1}{3}, \frac{7}{7}$.

. . . .

M, M, I, W, P, I, M, M, P, I

---

55. A mixed number may be changed to an improper fraction as follows: $4\frac{5}{8} = 4 + \frac{5}{8} = \frac{32}{8} + \frac{5}{8} = \frac{37}{8}$. Complete the following: $3\frac{9}{10} = 3 + \frac{9}{10} = \frac{30}{10} + \frac{9}{10} = $ _____ ; $4\frac{2}{5} = 4 + \frac{2}{5} = $ _____ ; $7\frac{1}{12} = $ _____ .

. . . .

$$3\tfrac{9}{10} = \frac{39}{10}; \quad 4\tfrac{2}{5} = \frac{20}{5} + \frac{2}{5} = \frac{22}{5}; \quad 7\tfrac{1}{12} = \frac{84}{12} + \frac{1}{12} = \frac{85}{12}$$

---

56. Change the following mixed numbers to improper fractions: $2\tfrac{1}{5}$, $5\tfrac{1}{12}$, $6\tfrac{1}{2}$, $11\tfrac{2}{3}$, $100\tfrac{5}{8}$.

. . . .

$$\frac{11}{5}, \frac{61}{12}, \frac{13}{2}, \frac{35}{3}, \frac{805}{8}$$

Just for fun, try this on a patient: Two volumes of a novel are standing side by side, in order, on a shelf, Volume I to the left of Volume II. If each cover is $\tfrac{1}{6}$ inch thick and each book without the cover is 1 inch thick, what is the distance between page 1 of Volume I and the last page of Volume II?*

. . . .

$\dfrac{1}{3}$ inch

When books stand in the customary fashion on a bookshelf, the first page of Volume I is on the right-hand side of the book and the last page of Volume II is on the left-hand side of the book. Therefore, only the covers are between page 1 of Volume I and the last page of Volume II. The covers together measure $\tfrac{1}{6}$ inch $+ \tfrac{1}{6}$ inch $= \tfrac{2}{6}$ inch or $\tfrac{1}{3}$ inch.

---

*See Jack Frohlichstein, *Mathematical Fun, Games and Puzzles*, Dover, New York, 1962, p. 76.

57. Complete the following table by filling in numbers equivalent to the given number on each line. For example, the first line is completed by filling in "1" in the column labeled "whole number."

Whole Number	Proper Fraction	Improper Fraction	Mixed Number
		$^{11}/_{11}$	
		$^{13}/_{5}$	
			$2^{1}/_{9}$
6			
			$5^{3}/_{10}$
			$3^{5}/_{8}$
		$^{33}/_{11}$	

. . . .

$\dfrac{13}{5} = 2^{3}/_{5}$, a mixed number

$2^{1}/_{9} = \dfrac{19}{9}$, an improper fraction

$6 = \dfrac{36}{6}$, an improper fraction (other possibilities include $\dfrac{6}{1}$, $\dfrac{12}{2}$, $\dfrac{60}{10}$, etc.)

$5^{3}/_{10} = \dfrac{53}{10}$, an improper fraction

$3^{5}/_{8} = \dfrac{29}{8}$, an improper fraction

$\dfrac{33}{11} = 3$, a whole number

58. The value of every _____ fraction is less than 1.

. . . .

proper (See Frame 45)

59. The value of every improper fraction with a numerator equal to the denominator is _____ .

. . . .

1   (See Frame 47)

60. The value of every mixed number is (less than/equal to/greater than) 1.

. . . .

greater than   *A mixed number is the sum of a whole number and a fraction.*

61. The value of every _____ fraction is less than 1; the value of every _____ fraction is greater than or equal to 1.

. . . .

The value of every proper fraction is less than 1; the value of every improper fraction is greater than or equal to 1.

62. Define proper fraction, improper fraction, and mixed number.

. . . .

See page 25, Item 5

SUMMARY

1. What is a fraction or simple ratio? A fraction or simple ratio is a symbol representing one or more of the equal parts into which a whole quantity or several whole quantities have been subdivided.

   Example: $\frac{3}{8}$ represents 3 of 8 equal parts into which a quantity has been divided.

2. What are the terms of a fraction? The denominator and numerator are the terms of a fraction. The denominator is the bottom number; the numerator is the top number. The denominator is the total number of equal subdivisions of the whole; the numerator is the number of subdivisions selected.

   Example: Given $\frac{3}{8}$, 3 is the numerator and 8 is the denominator.

3. How may the value of a fraction be increased? The value of a fraction may be increased by increasing its numerator or decreasing its denominator.

   Example: Suppose a fraction is needed with a value larger than $\frac{2}{5}$.

   Increase the numerator: $\frac{3}{5}$ is larger than $\frac{2}{5}$. Decrease the denominator: $\frac{2}{3}$ is also larger than $\frac{2}{5}$.

4. How are fractions added (or subtracted)? When the denominators are the same, add (or subtract) the numerators and retain the same denominator.

   Examples: $\frac{3}{5} + \frac{1}{5} = \frac{4}{5}$ $\frac{3}{5} - \frac{1}{5} = \frac{2}{5}$

5. Describe proper and improper fractions. A proper fraction is a fraction whose numerator is less than its denominator; its value is less than 1. A fraction whose numerator and denominator are equal to each other is an *improper fraction* with the value 1. A fraction with numerator greater than denominator is an *improper fraction* equivalent to a *mixed number*, the sum of a whole number and a proper fraction.

   Examples: $\frac{3}{5}$ is a proper fraction; its value is less than 1. But $\frac{5}{5}$ is an improper fraction; its value is equal to 1. Also, $\frac{9}{5}$ is an improper fraction; its value is equal to the mixed number $1\frac{4}{5}$.

EXERCISES FOR EXTRA PRACTICE

1. For each pair of fractions given below, state which are the numerators (N) and which are the denominators (D). Then select the larger fraction.

(a) $\dfrac{6}{13}, \dfrac{6}{11}$ (b) $\dfrac{2}{5}, \dfrac{3}{5}$ (c) $\dfrac{7}{11}, \dfrac{7}{15}$ (d) $\dfrac{35}{100}, \dfrac{11}{100}$

(e) $\dfrac{6}{14}, \dfrac{6}{10}$ (f) $\dfrac{8}{3}, \dfrac{8}{20}$ (g) $\dfrac{5}{7}, \dfrac{4}{7}$ (h) $\dfrac{23}{50}, \dfrac{38}{50}$

2. Carry out the operation indicated and express the result as a proper fraction, a whole number, or a mixed number.

(a) $\dfrac{3}{5} + \dfrac{2}{5} =$ (b) $\dfrac{5}{8} - \dfrac{2}{8} =$ (c) $\dfrac{11}{5} + \dfrac{2}{5} =$

(d) $\dfrac{2}{25}$ (e) $\dfrac{3}{100}$ (f) $\dfrac{9}{50}$ (g) $\dfrac{3}{10}$

$+ \dfrac{4}{25}$ $+ \dfrac{8}{100}$ $- \dfrac{2}{50}$ $+ \dfrac{7}{10}$

(h) $\dfrac{11}{20}$ (i) $\dfrac{99}{100}$ (j) $\dfrac{31}{50}$ (k) $\dfrac{175}{100}$

$+ \dfrac{13}{20}$ $- \dfrac{37}{100}$ $+ \dfrac{49}{50}$ $+ \dfrac{90}{100}$

3. (a) A 400-volume medical library contains 37 volumes on pharmacology and 40 volumes on obstetrics. After all the books on obstetrics are removed from the library, what is the ratio of pharmacology volumes to the total number of volumes?

(b) Make up your own example of a ratio whose denominator is two units more than its numerator.

(c) $^{15}\!/_{32}$ and $^{11}\!/_{32}$ are fractions with the same_____. Which fraction has the greater value? Explain.

(d) Which is greater, $^{3}\!/_{4}$ grain or $^{3}\!/_{7}$ grain?

(e) Give an example of a ratio that is greater than $^{1}\!/_{4}$ and has the same numerator as $^{1}\!/_{4}$.

(f) A dosage of $^{1}\!/_{9}$ grain of drug B is fatal. Give an example of a smaller dosage.

. . . .

Answers

1. (a) N = 6; D = 13, 11; $\dfrac{6}{11}$ (b) N = 2, 3; D = 5; $\dfrac{3}{5}$

   (c) N = 7; D = 11, 15; $\dfrac{7}{11}$ (d) N = 35, 11; D = 100; $\dfrac{35}{100}$

   (e) N = 6; D = 14, 10; $\dfrac{6}{10}$ (f) N = 8; D = 3; 20; $\dfrac{8}{3}$

   (g) N = 5, 4; D = 7; $\dfrac{5}{7}$ (h) N = 23; 38; D = 50; $\dfrac{38}{50}$

2. (a) 1   (b) $\dfrac{3}{8}$ (c) $2\dfrac{3}{5}$ (d) $\dfrac{6}{25}$ (e) $\dfrac{11}{100}$

   (f) $\dfrac{7}{50}$ (g) 1   (h) $1\dfrac{4}{20}$ or $1\dfrac{1}{5}$ (i) $\dfrac{62}{100}$ or $\dfrac{31}{50}$

   (j) $1\dfrac{30}{50}$ or $1\dfrac{3}{5}$ (k) $2\dfrac{65}{100}$ or $2\dfrac{13}{20}$

3. (a) $\dfrac{\text{number of pharmacology volumes}}{\text{total number of volumes}} = \dfrac{37}{400-40} = \dfrac{37}{360}$

   (b) Here are some possible answers: $\frac{1}{3}$, $\frac{2}{4}$, $\frac{3}{5}$, and so on.

   (c) The fractions have the same *denominator*. The total number of equal parts of a given object or collection, 32, is the same for each fraction, but the number of parts selected is greater in the first fraction (15). Therefore, $^{15}\!/_{32}$ represents a bigger portion of the whole than $^{11}\!/_{32}$.

   (d) $\frac{3}{4}$, since 3 of 4 subdivisions of a grain must each be greater than 3 of 7 subdivisions of a grain. The smaller the number of subdivisions, the greater each part must be.

   (e) $\dfrac{1}{3}$ or $\dfrac{1}{2}$

   (f) $\dfrac{1}{10}$, $\dfrac{1}{11}$, $\dfrac{1}{12}$, etc.

INVENTORY

The set of exercises below will show you whether you are already an expert or whether you need a little more practice. If you do need more practice, the numbers next to the answers on page 29 will direct you to the particular frames that should receive your special attention. Answer the following questions. If you have no errors you are an expert and are ready to advance to the next section. Otherwise, study the relevant frames and then work out the Proficiency Gauge on page 1.

1. An ounce is divided into 480 grains. What fractional part of the ounce is 17 grains?

2. If 2 ounces of a solution are poured into a bottle that already contains 5 ounces of the solution, what part of the total quantity was freshly poured?

3. Write a fraction in which the numerator is 2 units smaller than the denominator.

4. Which is greater, $\dfrac{1}{9}$ or $\dfrac{1}{10}$?

5. Which fraction represents the smallest quantity? $\dfrac{7}{10}, \dfrac{3}{7}, \dfrac{3}{10}$.

6. Add: $\dfrac{7}{11} + \dfrac{2}{11} + \dfrac{1}{11}$.

7. Subtract: $\dfrac{11}{17} - \dfrac{3}{17}$.

8. Is $\dfrac{91}{54}$ a proper fraction? Why?

9. Change $\dfrac{10}{7}$ to a mixed number.

10. Change $5\frac{2}{3}$ to an improper fraction.

11. Circle the improper fractions in the following list and change them to mixed numbers or whole numbers: $\dfrac{2}{3}, \dfrac{9}{5}, \dfrac{49}{7}, \dfrac{4}{7}, \dfrac{27}{8}, \dfrac{6}{6}$.

. . . .

Answers

1. $\frac{17}{480}$ (Frames 1—5)

2. $\frac{2}{7}$ (Frame 6)

3. $\frac{1}{3}, \frac{2}{4}, \frac{3}{5}, \frac{4}{6}, \frac{5}{7}$, etc. (Frames 7—12)

4. $\frac{1}{9}$ (Frames 16—28)

5. $\frac{3}{10}$ (Frames 16—28)

6. $\frac{10}{11}$ (Frames 29—33)

7. $\frac{8}{17}$ (Frame 33)

8. No; the numerator is greater than the denominator. (Frames 39—45)

9. $1\frac{3}{7}$ (Frames 51—52)

10. $\frac{17}{3}$ (Frames 55—57)

11. $\left(\frac{9}{5}\right) = 1\frac{4}{5}, \left(\frac{49}{7}\right) = 7, \left(\frac{27}{8}\right) = 3\frac{3}{8}, \left(\frac{6}{6}\right) = 1$ (Frames 55—57)

Reminder: If you made any errors, study the relevant frames and then work out the Proficiency Gauge. If you made no errors, proceed to Section 2.

COMMON FRACTIONS
SIMPLIFICATION, ADDITION, AND SUBTRACTION

In this section we discuss material that will enable the student to:

1. Know what is meant by "equivalent" fractions and how to recognize them and find fractions that are equivalent to a given fraction.

2. Simplify fractions.

3. Add and subtract fractions with unlike denominators.

PROFICIENCY GAUGE

It is possible that you do not need to review these topics. To gauge your proficiency, work out the following exercises. Uncover the printed answers only after you have answered all the questions. If you have made no errors, go right ahead to Section 3.

1. Find a fraction with denominator 30 that is equivalent to $\frac{8}{10}$.

2. Find a fraction with denominator 5 that is equivalent to $\frac{33}{165}$.

3. Simplify $\frac{45}{54}$ as much as possible.

4. Add: $\frac{2}{3} + \frac{2}{9}$.

5. Add: $\frac{7}{12} + \frac{2}{15}$.

6. Add: $7\frac{1}{4} + 2\frac{3}{5}$.

7. Subtract: $\frac{9}{10} - \frac{1}{6}$.

8. Subtract: $3\frac{7}{8} - 1\frac{5}{6}$.

9. Find x if $\frac{6}{x} = \frac{3}{7}$.

. . . .

Answers

1. $\dfrac{24}{30}$

2. $\dfrac{1}{5}$

3. $\dfrac{5}{6}$

4. $\dfrac{8}{9}$

5. $\dfrac{43}{60}$

6. $9\frac{17}{20}$

7. $\dfrac{22}{30}$ or $\dfrac{11}{15}$

8. $2\frac{1}{24}$ or $\dfrac{49}{24}$

9. 14

If you have made errors, go to Frame 63. Otherwise, go on to Section 3.

Read the instructions beginning on page 3 if you have not already done so.

Equivalent Fractions

If the numerator and denominator of a fraction are multiplied by the same number (not zero), the value of the fraction is unchanged. This fact enables us to find useful alternative forms for a given fraction.

---

63. When you exchange a half-dollar coin for quarters, how many quarters do you receive? Of course, 1 half-dollar = 2 quarters. Considering these coins as fractions of a dollar, $\frac{1}{2}$ dollar = $\frac{2}{?}$ dollar.

. . . .

$\frac{1}{2}$ dollar = $\frac{2}{4}$ dollar

---

64. A doctor prescribes $\frac{3}{4}$ grain aspirin for Baby Verasick. He has trouble swallowing tablets, so his mother breaks up the tablet into 8 little pieces and gives him enough to amount to $\frac{6}{8}$ grain. Has he received the correct amount?

. . . .

yes, $\frac{3}{4} = \frac{6}{8}$ *Three grains chosen from 4 grains is equivalent to 6 grains chosen from 8 grains.*

---

65. The pancake was divided into 3 equal portions. The shaded area represents what the patient has eaten. What fractional part of the pancake has he eaten? If the pancake had been divided into 6 equal portions, *how many portions* would be equivalent to $\frac{2}{3}$ pancake?

. . . .

$\frac{2}{3}$, 4 portions

---

66. Refer to previous frame. The patient has eaten $\frac{2}{3}$ of the pancake (cut in thirds). If the cake had been cut in sixths, he would have eaten 4 portions. Therefore, $\frac{2}{3}$ pancake is (more than/equivalent to/less than) $\frac{4}{6}$ pancake.

. . . .

equivalent to, i.e., $\frac{2}{3} = \frac{4}{6}$ *Eating 2 of 3 equal portions of a pancake is equivalent to eating 4 of 6 portions of the same pancake.*

---

67. $\frac{1}{2}$ grain = $\frac{2}{4}$ grain = $\frac{?}{8}$ grain.

. . . .

$$\frac{1}{2} = \frac{2}{4} = \frac{4}{8}$$

---

68. When the denominator is multiplied by two, then the numerator must be _____ _____ if the fractions are to be equivalent.

. . . .

multiplied by two

---

69. $\frac{2}{3} = \frac{6}{9} = \frac{?}{27}$; in each case, an equivalent fraction was found by multiplying both numerator and denominator by _____.

. . . .

$\frac{2}{3} = \frac{6}{9} = \frac{18}{27}$; multiplying both numerator and denominator by 3

---

70. $\frac{5}{7} = \frac{?}{35}$; if the denominator has been *multiplied* by _____ , then the numerator should be _____ by _____ to produce an equivalent fraction.

. . . .

$\frac{5}{7} = \frac{25}{35}$; if the denominator has been *multiplied* by 5, then the numerator should be *multiplied* by 5

---

71. $\frac{6}{11} = \frac{?}{33}$; if the denominator has been multiplied by 3, the new numerator will be found by _____ the old numerator by _____.

. . . .

$\frac{6}{11} = \frac{18}{33}$; if the denominator has been multiplied by 3, the new numerator will be found by *multiplying* the old numerator by 3

---

72. Find a fraction that is equivalent to $\frac{5}{12}$ but has denominator 48. (Multiply numerator and denominator of $\frac{5}{12}$ by _____.)

. . . .

$$\frac{5}{12} = \frac{20}{48}; \ 4 \qquad\qquad \frac{5}{12} = \frac{5 \times 4}{12 \times 4} = \frac{20}{48}$$

72a.

Find a ratio that is equivalent to $\frac{7}{11}$ and has a numerator of 42. (Multiply numerator and denominator of $\frac{7}{11}$ by _____.)

. . . .

$$\frac{7}{11} = \frac{42}{66}; \ 6$$

---

73. **Fundamental Principle of Fractions**
If the numerator and denominator of a given fraction or ratio are multiplied by the same number, the resulting new fraction or ratio is (greater than/equal to/less than) the given fraction.

. . . .

equal to

---

74. Write $\frac{8}{10}$ as a fraction with a denominator of 30.

. . . .

$$\frac{24}{30} \qquad\qquad \frac{8}{10} = \frac{8 \times 3}{10 \times 3} = \frac{24}{30}$$

---

75. Find a fraction that is equivalent to $\frac{5}{6}$ and has a denominator of 24.

. . . .

$$\frac{20}{24} \qquad\qquad \frac{5}{6} = \frac{5 \times 4}{6 \times 4} = \frac{20}{24}$$

76. Find a ratio with a denominator of 21 that is equivalent to $^2/_7$.

. . . .

$\frac{6}{21}$ (Multiply numerator and denominator of $\frac{2}{7}$ by 3.)

76a.

Find a ratio with a denominator of 12 that is equivalent to $^2/_3$.

. . . .

$\frac{8}{12}$ $\frac{2}{3} = \frac{2 \times 4}{3 \times 4} = \frac{8}{12}$

77. Find a fraction with a numerator of 6 that is equivalent to $^2/_5$.

. . . .

$\frac{6}{15}$ *Since 6 (the new numerator) is 3 × 2 (the old numerator), then the new denominator is 3 × 5 (the old denominator.)*

77a.

Find a fraction with a numerator of 100 that is equivalent to $^5/_9$.

. . . .

$\frac{100}{180}$ $\frac{5}{9} = \frac{5 \times 20}{9 \times 20} = \frac{100}{180}$

78. Find x if $\frac{x}{12} = \frac{2}{3}$.

. . . .

$x = 8$ *Since 12 = 4 × 3, then x = 4 × 2.*

78a.

Find x if $\dfrac{x}{10} = \dfrac{1}{5}$.

. . . .

$x = 2$ *Since 10 = 2 × 5, then x = 2 × 1.*

79. Find x if $\dfrac{48}{x} = \dfrac{8}{9}$.

. . . .

$x = 54$ *Since 48 = 6 × 8, then x = 6 × 9.*

79a.

Find x if $\dfrac{1}{6} = \dfrac{x}{30}$.

. . . .

$x = 5$ *Since 30 = 5 × 6, then x = 5 × 1.*

80. $\dfrac{2}{3} = \dfrac{?}{21}$; $\dfrac{5}{8} = \dfrac{?}{72}$; $\dfrac{7}{9} = \dfrac{28}{?}$.

. . . .

$\dfrac{2}{3} = \dfrac{14}{21}$; $\dfrac{5}{8} = \dfrac{45}{72}$; $\dfrac{7}{9} = \dfrac{28}{36}$

80a.

Write $\frac{7}{9}$ as a fraction with 54 as the denominator.

. . . .

$\dfrac{42}{54}$ $\dfrac{7}{9} = \dfrac{7 \times 6}{9 \times 6} = \dfrac{42}{54}$

81. You have been using the fundamental principle of fractions. State that principle. Check with page 49, Item 1.

Simplifying Fractions or Ratios

If the numerator and denominator of a fraction are divided by the same number (not zero), the value of the fraction is unchanged.

---

82. $^{100}/_{12} = {}^?/_3$. Let $^{100}/_{12}$ be the original fraction. The denominator of the new equivalent fraction is 3. By what do you divide 12 to get the new denominator, 3? Therefore, by what will you divide 100 to find the new numerator?

. . . .

$^{100}/_{12} = {}^{25}/_3$; 12 is divided by 4 to get the denominator 3 and therefore 100 should be divided by 4 to find the numerator of the equivalent simpler fraction.

---

83. Find a fraction whose numerator is 7 and which is equivalent to $^{56}/_{16}$; that is, $^{56}/_{16} = {}^7/_?$.

. . . .

$$\frac{56}{16} = \frac{7}{2}$$

The given numerator, 56, divided by 8 is the new numerator, 7. The given denominator, 16, divided by 8 is the new denominator, 2.

---

84. $\dfrac{38}{8} = \dfrac{?}{4}$.

. . . .

$$\frac{38}{8} = \frac{19}{4}$$

84a.

Find x if $\dfrac{36}{15} = \dfrac{x}{5}$.

. . . .

$x = 12$

Since 5 is 15 ÷ 3, x is 36 ÷ 3.

---

85. Find x if $\dfrac{x}{3} = \dfrac{49}{21}$.

$x = 7$ *Since 3 = 21 ÷ 7, x = 49 ÷ 7.*

85a.

Find x if $\dfrac{x}{11} = \dfrac{100}{22}$.

. . . .

$x = 50$

---

86. Find a fraction that is equivalent to $^{20}/_{48}$ but has a denominator of 12. (Divide the numerator and denominator by _____.)

. . . .

$\dfrac{20}{48} = \dfrac{5}{12}$; 4 $\dfrac{20}{48} = \dfrac{20 \div 4}{48 \div 4} = \dfrac{5}{12}$

86a.

Find a ratio that is equivalent to $^{66}/_{42}$ but has a denominator of 7. (Divide the numerator and denominator by _____.)

. . . .

$\dfrac{66}{42} = \dfrac{11}{7}$; 6 $\dfrac{66}{42} = \dfrac{66 \div 6}{42 \div 6} = \dfrac{11}{7}$

---

87. If the numerator and denominator of a given fraction are each divided by the same constant, the resulting fraction is (less than/equal to/greater than) the given fraction.

. . . .

equal to

---

88. Complete the following fractions: $\dfrac{12}{15} = \dfrac{4}{?}, \dfrac{?}{40} = \dfrac{2}{5}, \dfrac{36}{132} = \dfrac{?}{11}$.

. . . .

$\dfrac{12}{15} = \dfrac{4}{5}$

Since 4 is the result of dividing 12 by 3, divide 15 by 3 also.

$\dfrac{16}{40} = \dfrac{2}{5}$

Since 40 is the result of multiplying 5 by 8, multiply 2 by 8 also.

$\dfrac{36}{132} = \dfrac{3}{11}$

Since 11 is the result of dividing 132 by 12, divide 36 by 12 also.

88a.

Complete the following fractions: $\dfrac{6}{21} = \dfrac{?}{7}$, $\dfrac{6}{21} = \dfrac{24}{?}$, $\dfrac{?}{12} = \dfrac{3}{36}$.

. . . .

$\dfrac{6}{21} = \dfrac{2}{7}$

Since 7 is the result of dividing 21 by 3, divide 6 by 3 also.

$\dfrac{6}{21} = \dfrac{24}{84}$

Since 24 is the result of multiplying 6 by 4, multiply 21 by 4 also.

$\dfrac{1}{12} = \dfrac{3}{36}$

Since 12 is the result of dividing 36 by 3, divide 3 by 3 also.

---

89. $\dfrac{1000}{5750} = \dfrac{?}{575} = \dfrac{?}{115} = \dfrac{4}{?}$. Which is more likely to be convenient, $\dfrac{1000}{5750}$ or $\dfrac{4}{23}$?

. . . .

$\dfrac{1000}{5750} = \dfrac{100}{575} = \dfrac{20}{115} = \dfrac{4}{23}$

The numerator and denominator of $^{1000}/_{5750}$ may be divided by 10 to obtain $^{100}/_{575}$; then the numerator and denominator of $^{100}/_{575}$; may be divided by 5 to obtain $^{20}/_{115}$; repeating the process yields $^{4}/_{23}$.

$\dfrac{4}{23}$ is more convenient

Generally, the fraction with the smaller numerator and denominator is easier to deal with. Therefore we reduce numerators and denominators whenever feasible.

---

90. The fraction $^{90}/_{420}$ may be simplified by dividing the numerator and denominator by the same number. It is clear that 90 and 420 are both evenly divisible by 10 and what other number?

. . . .

3

91. Simplify $^{90}/_{420}$ by dividing the numerator and denominator by 30.

. . . .

$\dfrac{3}{14}$

Since 3 and 14 are not divisible by any whole number, $^3/_{14}$ cannot be simplified. ($^3/_{14}$ has been "reduced to lowest terms.")

---

92. Simplify $^{385}/_{1225}$ as much as possible. (Reduce to lowest terms.)

. . . .

Divide 385 and 1225 by any whole number that divides both the numerator and denominator evenly. Repeat the process with the simplified fraction until the numerator and denominator can no longer be divided evenly.

Answer: $\dfrac{11}{35}$

385 and 1225 are clearly both divisible by 5. Therefore $^{385}/_{1225} = {}^{77}/_{245}$. Now 77 and 245 are both divisible by 7. Therefore $^{77}/_{245} = {}^{11}/_{35}$. Since 11 and 35 are not both divisible by any whole number, $^{11}/_{35}$ cannot be simplified.

92a.

Simplify $\dfrac{520}{140}$.

. . . .

$\dfrac{520}{140} = \dfrac{52}{14} = \dfrac{26}{7}$

---

93. Simplify $\dfrac{18}{12}, \dfrac{333}{3000}, \dfrac{21}{70}$.

. . . .

$\dfrac{18}{12} = \dfrac{3}{2}; \quad \dfrac{333}{3000} = \dfrac{111}{1000}; \quad \dfrac{21}{70} = \dfrac{3}{10}$

94. Complete the sentence: Simplification of fractions means _____

_____ .

. . . .

Check with page 49 Item 2.

Addition and Subtraction of Fractions With Unlike Denominators

Change the fractions to equivalent fractions with like denominators. Then add or subtract the numerators and keep the denominator.

95. Lisa, a newborn infant, drank $\frac{1}{2}$ ounce of formula at the first feeding and $\frac{3}{4}$ ounce of formula at the second feeding. The doctor inquires about Lisa's total consumption in the two feedings, so the nurse must calculate $\frac{1}{2} + \frac{3}{4}$. It is easy to add fractions when the denominators are alike. Therefore, let us change $\frac{1}{2}$ to an equivalent fraction with denominator 4 and add the result to $\frac{3}{4}$.

. . . .

$$\frac{1}{2} = \frac{2}{4}$$

$$\frac{2}{4} + \frac{3}{4} = \frac{5}{4}$$

$$\frac{5}{4} = 1\frac{1}{4} \text{ ounces}$$

96. If the baby had drunk $\frac{2}{3}$ ounce and $\frac{3}{5}$ ounce, what would her total consumption have been? (Change both fractions to equivalent fractions with denominator 15.)

$$\frac{2}{3} = \frac{?}{15}; \ \frac{3}{5} = \frac{?}{15}; \ \frac{2}{3} + \frac{3}{5} = \frac{?}{15}$$

. . . .

$$\frac{2}{3} = \frac{10}{15}; \ \frac{3}{5} = \frac{9}{15}; \ \frac{2}{3} + \frac{3}{5} = \frac{19}{15} \ \text{(or } 1\frac{4}{15} \text{ ounces)}$$

96a.

If Lisa drank $\frac{4}{5}$ ounce and then $\frac{5}{8}$ ounce, how much did she drink in all?

. . . .

$1^{17}/_{40}$ $\qquad$ $\dfrac{4}{5} + \dfrac{5}{8}$ *must be changed to* $\dfrac{32}{40} + \dfrac{25}{40} = \dfrac{57}{40}$

---

97. In a rare quiet moment, the pharmacist had a chance to consolidate the drug sup-
plies. He emptied the contents of three partially filled flasks of drug *A* into one
large flask and labeled the resulting quantity appropriately. What number of
ounces would he have written on the label if the first flask contained $2\frac{1}{4}$ ounces,
the second contained $3\frac{1}{8}$ ounces, and the third $1\frac{1}{2}$ ounces?

. . . .

$6\frac{7}{8}$

(1) You may work with the whole numbers first: *2 + 3 + 1 = 6.*

(2) Then $\dfrac{1}{4} + \dfrac{1}{8} + \dfrac{1}{2}$ *must be changed to*

$\dfrac{2}{8} + \dfrac{1}{8} + \dfrac{4}{8} = \dfrac{7}{8}$.

(3) All together, there were $6\frac{7}{8}$ ounces of
the drug.

97a.

Add: $1\frac{1}{2}$ ounces + $2\frac{7}{8}$ ounces + $5\frac{1}{4}$ ounces.

. . . .

$9\frac{5}{8}$

(1) First add the whole numbers:
1 + 2 + 5 = 8.

(2) Then add the fractions: $\dfrac{1}{2} + \dfrac{7}{8} + \dfrac{1}{4}$

must be changed to $\dfrac{4}{8} + \dfrac{7}{8} + \dfrac{2}{8} = \dfrac{13}{8} =$

$1\frac{5}{8}$.

(3) All together, $8 + 1\frac{5}{8} = 9\frac{5}{8}$.

---

98. Add: $\dfrac{25}{3} + \dfrac{3}{2} + \dfrac{1}{5}$. (All three fractions must be changed to equivalent fractions

with the same denominator. The denominators 3, 2, and 5 all divide evenly into
what numbers?)

. . . .

$\dfrac{301}{30}$ or $10\frac{1}{30}$

(1) The denominators 3, 2, and 5 all divide evenly into 30, also into 60, also into 90, and so on. We use 30, the smallest of all the possibilities, for the new denominator.

(2) We change $\dfrac{25}{3}$ to $\dfrac{250}{30}$, $\dfrac{3}{2}$ to $\dfrac{45}{30}$, and $\dfrac{1}{5}$ to $\dfrac{6}{30}$.

(3) Then we can add: $\dfrac{250}{30} + \dfrac{45}{30} + \dfrac{6}{30} =$ $\dfrac{301}{30}$ or $10\frac{1}{30}$.

---

99. Add $\dfrac{3}{10} + \dfrac{2}{5} + \dfrac{5}{3}$ (the denominators 10, 5, and 3 all divide evenly into _____ .)

. . . .

$2\frac{11}{30}$

(1) The denominators 10, 5, and 3 all divide evenly into 30; also into 150; also into many other numbers. We use 30, the smallest of all the possibilities, for the new denominator.

(2) We change $\dfrac{3}{10}$ to $\dfrac{9}{30}$, $\dfrac{2}{5}$ to $\dfrac{12}{30}$, and $\dfrac{5}{3}$ to $\dfrac{50}{30}$.

(3) Then $\dfrac{9}{30} + \dfrac{12}{30} + \dfrac{50}{30} = \dfrac{71}{30}$ or $2\frac{11}{30}$.

99a.

Add: $\dfrac{2}{3} + \dfrac{7}{8} + \dfrac{5}{12}$.

. . . .

$1\frac{23}{24}$

We change $\dfrac{2}{3} + \dfrac{7}{8} + \dfrac{5}{12}$ to $\dfrac{16}{24} + \dfrac{21}{24} + \dfrac{10}{24} =$ $\dfrac{47}{24}$.

100. Add: $1\frac{3}{4} + 2\frac{5}{6}$.

. . . .

$4\frac{7}{12}$

(1) Add the fractions: $\frac{3}{4} + \frac{5}{6} = \frac{9}{12} + \frac{10}{12} =$

$\frac{19}{12} = 1\frac{7}{12}$.

(2) Add the whole numbers: 1 + 2 = 3.

(3) Combine the results: $3 + 1\frac{7}{12} = 4\frac{7}{12}$.

100a.

Add: $7\frac{1}{9} + 2\frac{5}{12}$.

. . . .

$9\frac{19}{36}$

7 + 2 = 9

$\frac{1}{9} + \frac{5}{12} = \frac{4}{36} + \frac{15}{36} = \frac{19}{36}$

Total: $9 + \frac{19}{36} = 9\frac{19}{36}$

Subtraction of Fractions With Unlike Denominators

101. The United States inspector has scheduled a visit and you are required to fill out an inventory of drugs on hand. There had been 32 ounces of boric acid and $3\frac{5}{8}$ ounces have been used up. How much is left? (Change 32 to a convenient mixed number, $31\frac{8}{8}$.)

. . . .

$28\frac{3}{8}$

(1) Think of 32 as $31\frac{8}{8}$.

(2) Subtract the fractions: $\frac{8}{8} - \frac{5}{8} = \frac{3}{8}$.

(3) Subtract the whole numbers: 31 − 3 = 28.

(4) Combine the totals: $28\frac{3}{8}$.

101a.

Find $15 - 2\frac{3}{16}$.

. . . .

$12\frac{13}{16}$

(1) *Change 15 to $14\frac{16}{16}$*

(2) *Then $14\frac{16}{16} - 2\frac{3}{16} = 12\frac{13}{16}$.*

102. The nurse spilled sterile water on the floor. The bottle had contained $4\frac{3}{4}$ ounces and now contains only $2\frac{1}{2}$ ounces. How much did she waste?

. . . .

$2\frac{1}{4}$ ounces

(1) *Change $\frac{1}{2}$ to $\frac{2}{4}$.*

(2) *Subtract the fractions: $\frac{3}{4} - \frac{2}{4} = \frac{1}{4}$.*

(3) *Subtract the whole numbers: $4 - 2 = 2$.*

(4) *Combine the results.*

102a.

Find $5\frac{7}{8} - 2\frac{3}{4}$.

. . . .

$3\frac{1}{8}$

(1) *Change $\frac{3}{4}$ to $\frac{6}{8}$.*

(2) *Subtract the fractions: $\frac{7}{8} - \frac{6}{8} = \frac{1}{8}$.*

(3) *Subtract the whole numbers: $5 - 2 = 3$.*

(4) *Combine the results: $3 + \frac{1}{8} = 3\frac{1}{8}$.*

103. Subtract: $8\frac{5}{9} - 2\frac{1}{12}$.

. . . .

$6^{17}/_{36}$

(1) Change $\frac{5}{9}$ to $\frac{20}{36}$; change $\frac{1}{12}$ to $\frac{3}{36}$.

(2) Subtract the fractions: $\frac{20}{36} - \frac{3}{36} = \frac{17}{36}$.

(3) Subtract the whole numbers: $8 - 2 = 6$.

(4) Combine the results: $6 + \frac{17}{36} = 6^{17}/_{36}$.

103a.

Subtract: $7^5/_6 - 3^1/_4$.

. . . .

$4^7/_{12}$

(1) Change $\frac{5}{6}$ to $\frac{10}{12}$; change $\frac{1}{4}$ to $\frac{3}{12}$.

(2) Then $7^5/_6 - 3^1/_4$ is equivalent to $7^{10}/_{12} - 3^3/_{12}$ or $4^7/_{12}$.

---

104. Find $7^1/_4 - 2^5/_8$.

. . . .

$4^5/_8$

(1) Change $7^1/_4$ to $7^2/_8$.

(2) Change 7 to $6^8/_8$.

(3) Thus $7^2/_8 = 6^{10}/_8$.

(4) Then $6^{10}/_8 - 2^5/_8 = 4^5/_8$.

104a.

Find $11^2/_3 - 2^{11}/_{12}$.

. . . .

$8^3/_4$

(1) Change $11^2/_3$ to $11^8/_{12}$.

(2) Change 11 to $10^{12}/_{12}$.

(3) Then $11^2/_3 = 10^{20}/_{12}$.

(4) Now we are ready to subtract: $11^2/_3 - 2^{11}/_{12} = 10^{20}/_{12} - 2^{11}/_{12} = 8^9/_{12}$ or $8^3/_4$.

104b.

Subtract $7\frac{4}{5}$ from $12\frac{1}{4}$.

. . . .

$4\frac{9}{20}$

(1) Change $7\frac{4}{5}$ to $7\frac{16}{20}$.

(2) Change $12\frac{1}{4}$ to $12\frac{5}{20}$.

(3) Then $12\frac{1}{4} - 7\frac{4}{5} = 12\frac{5}{20} - 7\frac{16}{20}$.

(4) Change $12\frac{5}{20}$ to $11\frac{25}{20}$.

(5) $11\frac{25}{20} - 7\frac{16}{20} = 4\frac{9}{20}$.

105. Complete: The important thing to remember about adding or subtracting fractions with unlike denominators is _____

_____ .

. . . .

Check with page 49, Item 3.

SUMMARY

1. To find a new fraction that is equivalent to a given fraction, multiply (or divide) the numerator and denominator by the same number (except zero).

   Examples: (a) Given $\dfrac{2}{3} = \dfrac{?}{15}$, note that $3 \times 5 = 15$. Then $\dfrac{2}{3} = \dfrac{2 \times 5}{3 \times 5}$.

   Thus $\dfrac{2}{3}$ is equivalent to $\dfrac{10}{15}$.

   (b) Given $\dfrac{20}{12} = \dfrac{?}{3}$, note that $12 \div 4 = 3$. Then $\dfrac{20}{12} = \dfrac{20 \div 4}{12 \div 4}$

   and $\dfrac{20}{12}$ is equivalent to $\dfrac{5}{3}$.

2. To simplify a fraction, find an equivalent fraction with a smaller numerator and denominator.

   Example: To simplify $\dfrac{10}{12}$, note that $\dfrac{10}{12} = \dfrac{5 \times 2}{6 \times 2}$. Thus $\dfrac{10}{12} = \dfrac{5}{6}$.

3. To add or subtract fractions with unlike denominators, first change them to fractions with like denominators.

   Example: $\dfrac{3}{8} + \dfrac{1}{6} = \dfrac{9}{24} + \dfrac{4}{24} = \dfrac{13}{24}$

EXERCISES FOR EXTRA PRACTICE

1. Complete the following fractions.

   (a) $\dfrac{2}{3} = \dfrac{?}{6}$ (b) $\dfrac{2}{5} = \dfrac{8}{?}$ (c) $\dfrac{3}{7} = \dfrac{?}{21}$ (d) $\dfrac{?}{50} = \dfrac{7}{10}$

   (e) $\dfrac{32}{?} = \dfrac{8}{25}$ (f) $\dfrac{45}{?} = \dfrac{9}{11}$ (g) $\dfrac{3}{20} = \dfrac{?}{100}$

2. Simplify the following fractions as much as possible.

   (a) $\dfrac{12}{150}$ (b) $\dfrac{50}{75}$ (c) $\dfrac{28}{44}$ (d) $\dfrac{20}{180}$ (e) $\dfrac{9}{51}$

3. Carry out the indicated operations and express the answer as a proper fraction or mixed number.

   (a) $\dfrac{3}{10} + \dfrac{2}{5}$ (b) $\dfrac{2}{3} + \dfrac{5}{12}$ (c) $\dfrac{3}{4} - \dfrac{2}{3}$ (d) $\dfrac{7}{12} - \dfrac{3}{10}$

   (e) $2\dfrac{7}{20} + 5\dfrac{3}{25}$ (f) $4\dfrac{3}{25} - 3\dfrac{1}{10}$ (g) $4\dfrac{8}{15} + 1\dfrac{3}{50}$ (h) $2\dfrac{99}{100} - \dfrac{3}{25}$

   (i) $3\dfrac{1}{10} - 2\dfrac{5}{8}$

. . . .

Answers

1. (a) $\dfrac{2}{3} = \dfrac{4}{6}$ (b) $\dfrac{2}{5} = \dfrac{8}{20}$ (c) $\dfrac{3}{7} = \dfrac{9}{21}$ (d) $\dfrac{35}{50} = \dfrac{7}{10}$

   (e) $\dfrac{32}{100} = \dfrac{8}{25}$ (f) $\dfrac{45}{55} = \dfrac{9}{11}$ (g) $\dfrac{3}{20} = \dfrac{15}{100}$

2. (a) $\dfrac{12}{150} = \dfrac{2}{25}$ (b) $\dfrac{2}{3}$ (c) $\dfrac{7}{11}$ (d) $\dfrac{1}{9}$ (e) $\dfrac{3}{17}$

3. (a) $\dfrac{7}{10}$ (b) $1\dfrac{1}{12}$ (c) $\dfrac{1}{12}$ (d) $\dfrac{17}{60}$ (e) $7\dfrac{47}{100}$

   (f) $1\dfrac{1}{50}$ (g) $5\dfrac{89}{150}$ (h) $2\dfrac{87}{100}$ (i) $\dfrac{19}{40}$

INVENTORY

Answer the following questions. If you have no errors, you are ready to advance to Section 3. If you have errors, study the relevant frames indicated below. Then go back to the Proficiency Gauge on page 31.

1. Find a fraction with a denominator of 24 that is equivalent to $\frac{5}{6}$.

2. Find a fraction with a denominator of 12 that is equivalent to $\frac{40}{96}$.

3. Simplify $\frac{42}{90}$ as much as possible.

4. Add: $\frac{2}{3} + \frac{1}{9}$.

5. Add: $\frac{7}{15} + \frac{5}{12}$.

6. Add: $7\frac{1}{4} + 2\frac{5}{6}$.

7. Subtract: $\frac{7}{12} - \frac{2}{15}$.

8. Subtract: $7\frac{1}{4} - 2\frac{3}{5}$.

9. Find x if $\frac{48}{x} = \frac{8}{9}$.

. . . .

Answers

1. $\frac{5}{6} = \frac{20}{24}$ (Frames 63—81)

2. $\frac{5}{12}$ (Frames (63—81)

3. $\frac{42}{90} = \frac{7}{15}$ (Frames 82—94)

4. $\frac{2}{3} + \frac{1}{9} = \frac{7}{9}$ (Frames 95—100)

5. $\frac{28}{60} + \frac{25}{60} = \frac{53}{60}$ (Frames 95—100)

6. $10\frac{1}{12}$ (Frames 95—100)

7. $\frac{27}{60} = \frac{9}{20}$ (Frames 101—102)

8. $4\frac{13}{20}$ (Frames 101—105)

9. 54 (Frames 63—81)

COMMON FRACTIONS
MULTIPLICATION
AND DIVISION

In this section, we cover material that will enable the student to:

1. Multiply and divide common fractions and mixed numbers by whole numbers, fractions, and mixed numbers, and simplify the results.

2. Solve verbal problems requiring the operations described above.

PROFICIENCY GAUGE

It is possible that you already know these topics. To gauge your proficiency, work out the following exercises. Uncover the printed answers only after you have answered all the questions. If you have no errors, skip ahead to Section 4.

1. Multiply: $\frac{5}{8} \times 9$.

2. Multiply: $\frac{2}{3} \times \frac{2}{5}$.

3. Multiply: $2\frac{3}{4} \times 3\frac{2}{7}$.

4. Multiply: $\frac{5}{8} \times \frac{4}{15}$.

5. Multiply: $\frac{4}{9} \times \frac{15}{16}$.

6. Multiply: $5\frac{1}{4} \times 1\frac{5}{7}$.

7. Divide: $\frac{1}{9} \div \frac{1}{2}$.

8. Divide: $\frac{3}{4} \div \frac{3}{8}$.

9. Divide: $1\frac{4}{5} \div 2\frac{1}{10}$

10. A flask of a certain solution contains $3\frac{1}{8}$ ounces of dextrose. How much dextrose will $2\frac{2}{5}$ flasks of this solution contain?

11. How many doses can be dispensed if $1\frac{4}{5}$ ounces are available and each dose requires $\frac{3}{20}$ ounce?

. . . .

Answers

1. $\frac{45}{8}$ or $5\frac{5}{8}$

2. $\frac{4}{15}$

3. $\frac{253}{28}$ or $9\frac{1}{28}$

4. $\frac{1}{6}$

5. $\frac{5}{12}$

6. 9

7. $\frac{2}{9}$

8. 2

9. $\frac{6}{7}$

10. $\frac{15}{2}$ or $7\frac{1}{2}$

11. 12 doses

Read the instructions on page 3 if you have not done so.

Multiplication of Fractions

Multiply numerators and multiply denominators. Simplify first if possible.

___

106. A very young child may be given a dose of $\frac{1}{4}$ of a 5-grain aspirin. When he grows a little older, he may have double the dose. The new dosage would be 2 aspirins, $\frac{1}{8}$ aspirin, or $\frac{2}{4}$ aspirin?

. . . .

$\frac{2}{4}$ aspirin $\qquad$ $\frac{1}{4}$ doubled $= 2 \times \frac{1}{4} = \frac{1}{4} + \frac{1}{4} = \frac{2}{4}$ (may be

reduced to $\frac{1}{2}$)

___

107. When the child is still older, he will be given triple the original dose of $\frac{1}{4}$ aspirin, which is _____ aspirin.

. . . .

$\frac{3}{4}$ $\qquad$ $\frac{1}{4}$ tripled $= 3 \times \frac{1}{4} = \frac{1}{4} + \frac{1}{4} + \frac{1}{4} = \frac{3}{4}$

___

108. How much is $5 \times \frac{1}{4}$?

. . . .

$\frac{5}{4}$ $\qquad$ $5 \times \frac{1}{4} = \frac{1}{4} + \frac{1}{4} + \frac{1}{4} + \frac{1}{4} + \frac{1}{4} = \frac{5}{4}$

___

108a.

Multiply: $7 \times \frac{1}{10}$.

. . . .

$\frac{7}{10}$

___

109. Seven flasks are standing on a shelf. Each contains $\frac{4}{5}$ quart of distilled water. How much distilled water is there all together?

. . . .

$5\frac{3}{5}$ quarts $7 \times \dfrac{4}{5} = \dfrac{28}{5} = 5\frac{3}{5}$ *quarts of distilled water*

---

110. Multiply: $3 \times \dfrac{9}{10}$.

. . . .

$\dfrac{27}{10} = 2\frac{7}{10}$

110a.

Multiply: $5 \times \dfrac{7}{12}$.

. . . .

$\dfrac{35}{12} = 2\frac{11}{12}$

---

111. You have been multiplying a whole number by a fraction. The whole number may be written as a fraction also: $3 \times \dfrac{1}{4}$ may be written as $\dfrac{3}{1} \times \dfrac{1}{4}$. The product is $\dfrac{3 \times 1}{1 \times 4} = \dfrac{3}{4}$. $5 \times \dfrac{1}{4}$ may be written as $\dfrac{5}{1} \times \dfrac{1}{4} = \dfrac{5 \times 1}{1 \times 4}$. The product is $\dfrac{5}{4}$. $7 \times \dfrac{1}{10}$ may be written as _____. The product is _____.

. . . .

$\dfrac{7}{1} \times \dfrac{1}{10} = \dfrac{7 \times 1}{1 \times 10} = \dfrac{7}{10}$

111a.

$7 \times \dfrac{4}{5}$ may be written as _____. The product is _____.

. . . .

$\dfrac{7}{1} \times \dfrac{4}{5} = \dfrac{28}{5}$ or $5\frac{3}{5}$

---

112. Write $7 \times \frac{5}{9}$ as a fraction times a fraction and find the product.

. . . .

$\frac{7}{1} \times \frac{5}{9} = \frac{35}{9}$ or $3\frac{8}{9}$

112a.

Multiply: $17 \times \frac{2}{59}$.

. . . .

$\frac{34}{59}$

$17 \times \frac{2}{59} = \frac{17}{1} \times \frac{2}{59} = \frac{34}{59}$

---

113. Write a rule for multiplying fractions.

. . . .

To multiply two fractions, multiply the numerators and multiply the denominators.

---

114. Find $\frac{3}{5} \times \frac{1}{4}$.

. . . .

$\frac{3}{5} \times \frac{1}{4} = \frac{3}{20}$

114a.

Find $\frac{3}{7} \times \frac{1}{10}$.

. . . .

$\frac{3}{7} \times \frac{1}{10} = \frac{3}{70}$

115. A tablet weighs $\frac{5}{7}$ ounce. What is the weight of two tablets? of $\frac{1}{3}$ tablet?

. . . .

$$2 \times \frac{5}{7} = \frac{10}{7} \text{ ounce;} \quad \frac{1}{3} \times \frac{5}{7} = \frac{5}{21} \text{ ounce}$$

116. A tablet weighs $\frac{5}{7}$ ounce. What is the weight of $\frac{3}{4}$ of the tablet?

. . . .

$\frac{15}{28}$ ounce $\frac{3}{4} \times \frac{5}{7} = \frac{15}{28}$

116a.

Knowing that $\frac{1}{20}$ ounce of arsenic will cause death, a member of the underworld obtained a vial containing $\frac{1}{4}$ ounce of arsenic and poured $\frac{1}{3}$ of it into his partner's tea. (He didn't want to waste any.) Did he use enough? Why?

. . . .

Yes. $\frac{1}{3} \times \frac{1}{4} = \frac{1}{12}$, which is greater than $\frac{1}{20}$.

117. Multiply: $\frac{4}{7} \times \frac{9}{11}$. Find the product of $\frac{2}{9} \times \frac{7}{10}$.

. . . .

$\frac{36}{77}$; $\frac{14}{90}$ (or $\frac{7}{45}$)

117a.

Multiply: $\frac{3}{4} \times \frac{5}{7}$.

. . . .

$\frac{15}{28}$

118. Given $\frac{2}{7}$ and $\frac{3}{7}$, the sum is _____ ; the product is _____.

. . . .

$\frac{2}{7} + \frac{3}{7} = \frac{5}{7}$ (See Frames 29–31); $\frac{2}{7} \times \frac{3}{7} = \frac{6}{49}$ (See Frame 113)

118a.

Find $\frac{1}{5} + \frac{3}{5}$; find $\frac{1}{5} \times \frac{3}{5}$.

. . . .

$\frac{1}{5} + \frac{3}{5} = \frac{4}{5}$; $\frac{1}{5} \times \frac{3}{5} = \frac{3}{25}$

---

119. $\frac{4}{15} \times \frac{7}{10} = \frac{4 \times 7}{15 \times 10}$, but do not multiply out yet. First simplify. Since 2 is a common divisor of the numerator and denominator, divide the numerator and denominator by 2. The problem then becomes $\frac{? \times 7}{15 \times ?}$, and the final product is _____.

. . . .

$\frac{14}{75}$

Did you divide the numerator and denominator by 2?

$$\frac{4}{15} \times \frac{7}{10} = \frac{^2\!\!4 \times 7}{15 \times 10_5} = \frac{2 \times 7}{15 \times 5} = \frac{14}{75}$$

119a.

Find $\frac{9}{11} \times \frac{5}{24}$.

. . . .

$\frac{9}{11} \times \frac{5}{24} = \frac{9 \times 5}{11 \times 24}$

$= \frac{15}{88}$

Divide the numerator and denominator by 3:

$$\frac{^3\!\!9 \times 5}{11 \times 24_8}$$

The product is $\frac{15}{88}$.

120. Multiply: $\frac{3}{4} \times \frac{2}{5} \times \frac{7}{15}$.

. . . .

$\frac{7}{50}$

The product is $\frac{3 \times 2 \times 7}{4 \times 5 \times 15}$. Did you notice that you could divide the numerator and denominator by 3?

$$\frac{^1\cancel{3} \times 2 \times 7}{4 \times 5 \times \cancel{15}_5}$$

Did you notice that you could divide the numerator and denominator by 2?

$$\frac{1 \times {}^1\cancel{2} \times 7}{_2\cancel{4} \times 5 \times 5} = \frac{7}{2 \times 25} = \frac{7}{50}$$

120a.

Multiply: $\frac{36}{49} \times 9 \times \frac{7}{24}$.

. . . .

$$\frac{^3\cancel{36} \times 9 \times \cancel{7}^1}{\cancel{49}_7 \times 1 \times \cancel{24}_2} = \frac{27}{14} = 1\,^{13}/_{14}$$

121. Find $5\frac{1}{9} \times \frac{27}{32}$.

. . . .

$$5\frac{1}{9} \times \frac{27}{32} = \frac{46}{9} \times \frac{27}{32} = \frac{^{23}\cancel{46} \times \cancel{27}^3}{_1\cancel{9} \times \cancel{32}_{16}} = \frac{69}{16} \text{ or } 4\,^5/_{16}$$

122. Find the sum and product of $3\frac{5}{6}$ and $1\frac{5}{16}$.

. . . .

To find the *sum:*

(a) Both fractions must have the same denominator. Therefore change $\frac{5}{6}$ to $\frac{40}{48}$ and $\frac{5}{16}$ to $\frac{15}{48}$.

(b) Add: $\frac{40}{48} + \frac{15}{48} = \frac{55}{48} = 1\frac{7}{48}$.

(c) Add: $3 + 1 + 1\frac{7}{48} = 5\frac{7}{48}$.

To find the *product:*

(a) Both mixed numbers should be changed to fractions: $3\frac{5}{6} = \frac{23}{6}$; $1\frac{5}{16} = \frac{21}{16}$.

(b) Multiply: $\frac{23}{6} \times \frac{21}{16} = \frac{23}{2\not{6}} \times \frac{\not{21}^{7}}{16} = \frac{23 \times 7}{2 \times 16} = \frac{161}{32}$.

---

123. One ounce of Dreerios cereal contains 112 calories. A box containing one serving of Dreerios contains $\frac{7}{8}$ ounces. How many calories are there per serving?

. . . .

$\frac{7}{_{1}\not{8}} \times \not{112}^{14} = 98$ calories

---

124. How many seconds are there in $5\frac{1}{4}$ hours?

. . . .

18,900 seconds

There are 60 seconds in 1 minute. There are 60 × 60 seconds in 60 minutes. There are 3600 seconds in 1 hour. There are 3600 × $5\frac{1}{4}$ seconds in $5\frac{1}{4}$ hours. $^{900}\not{3600} \times \frac{21}{\not{4}_{1}} = 18,900$ seconds.

124a.

How many seconds are there in $3\frac{1}{2}$ minutes?

. . . .

210 seconds

There are 60 seconds in 1 minute. There are 60 × $3\frac{1}{2}$ seconds in $3\frac{1}{2}$ minutes. $60 \times 3\frac{1}{2} = {}^{30}\not{60} \times \frac{7}{\not{2}_{1}} = 210$.

---

125. Each cup of batter weighs $3\frac{1}{2}$ ounces. What is the weight of $2\frac{2}{3}$ cups of batter?

. . . .

$9\frac{1}{3}$

The weight of 1 cup is $3\frac{1}{2}$ ounces. The weight of $2\frac{2}{3}$ cups is $2\frac{2}{3} \times 3\frac{1}{2}$ ounces.

$$2\frac{2}{3} \times 3\frac{1}{2} = \frac{\overset{4}{\cancel{8}}}{3} \times \frac{7}{\underset{1}{\cancel{2}}} = \frac{28}{3} \text{ or } 9\frac{1}{3}$$

125a.

What is the weight of $7\frac{1}{4}$ bars of chocolate if each bar weighs $1\frac{1}{3}$ ounces?

. . . .

$9\frac{2}{3}$

The weight of 1 bar is $1\frac{1}{3}$ ounces. The weight of $7\frac{1}{4}$ bars is $7\frac{1}{4} \times 1\frac{1}{3}$ ounces.

$$7\frac{1}{4} \times 1\frac{1}{3} = \frac{29}{\underset{1}{\cancel{4}}} \times \frac{\cancel{4}}{3} = \frac{29}{3} \text{ or } 9\frac{2}{3}$$

---

126. (a) What is the rule for multiplication of fractions?

(b) How may the multiplication be simplified when common divisors are present?

(c) What should be done as the first step in multiplying mixed numbers?

(d) If quantitative information q is given about one item, then similar quantitative information about n identical items can be found by_____.

. . . .

Check page 71, Items 1, 2, 3, 5.

Division of Fractions
Invert the divisor. Then multiply.

---

127. The doctor has ordered 4 tablets of a drug per day for a patient. If 8 tablets are left in stock, how many more days will the supply last? In answering this simple question, note the arithmetic process you use so that you may apply it to problems with fractions.

. . . .

2

> *Eight capsules must be divided into doses of 4 capsules each. There are $8 \div 4$ or $\dfrac{8}{4}$ or 2 such doses.*

---

128. The doctor next ordered 2 tablets per day for his patient. The patient has 8 tablets left. For how many more days will his supply last?

$8 \div 2 = \dfrac{8}{2} =$ _____

. . . .

4

$$\dfrac{8}{2} = 8 \div 2 = 4$$

> *Eight capsules must be divided into doses of 2 capsules each. There are 4 such doses.*

---

129. If a man has 8 tablets and must take $\frac{1}{2}$ tablet a day, his supply should last _____ how many days?

$8 \div \dfrac{1}{2} = \dfrac{8}{\frac{1}{2}} =$ _____ . This is the same as $8 \times$ _____ .

. . . .

16; 2

$$8 \div \dfrac{1}{2} = \dfrac{8}{\frac{1}{2}} = 16$$

> *In this case, 8 capsules are being divided up into doses of $\frac{1}{2}$ capsule each. There are 16 such doses.*

---

130. If a nurse's aide has 9 inches of adhesive tape and cuts the tape into pieces of length $\frac{1}{3}$ inch, how many pieces of tape will we have?

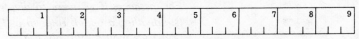

$9 \div \dfrac{1}{3} =$ _____ $=$ _____ . This is the same as

$9 \times$ _____ .

. . . .

27; 3

> *9 inches are being divided into pieces of length $\frac{1}{3}$ inches.*
> $$9 \div \dfrac{1}{3} = \dfrac{9}{\frac{1}{3}} = 9 \times 3 = 27$$

131. $\dfrac{10}{1/_5}$ is the same as 10 × _____ .

. . . .

5   *If 10 inches were divided into pieces of*
                                     length $\frac{1}{5}$ inch, there would be 50 pieces.

131a.

$\dfrac{7}{1/_9}$ is the same as 7 × _____ .

. . . .

9

131b.

$\dfrac{6}{1/_7}$ is the same as 6 × _____ .

. . . .

7

---

132. To divide any number by $\dfrac{1}{x}$, multiply that number by _____ .

. . . .

x   *For instance, if we were to divide 6 by $\frac{1}{3}$*
                                     (subdividing a 6-inch ruler into $\frac{1}{3}$-inch sec-
                                     tions) we would multiply 6 × 3. There are
                                     18 subdivisions.

132a.

To divide any number by $\frac{1}{6}$, multiply that number by _____ .

. . . .

6

---

133. As a graduation gift Nurse Susan Dear received a 5-ounce vial of Arpege. If Susan uses $\frac{1}{12}$ ounce on every date, for how many dates will the perfume last?

· · · · · · · · · · · ·

60

5 ounces must be divided into portions of $\frac{1}{12}$ ounce each. How many portions are there?

$$5 \div \frac{1}{12} = 5 \times 12 = 60$$

133a.

$$10 \div \frac{1}{2} = \underline{\hspace{2cm}}.$$

· · · · · · · · · · · ·

20

$$10 \div \frac{1}{2} = 10 \times 2 = 20$$

134. Pieces of tape of length $\frac{2}{3}$ inch are to be cut from 6 inches of tape. Count off how many pieces of tape there would be.

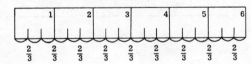

$$6 \div \frac{2}{3} = \underline{\hspace{2cm}} = 6 \times \underline{\hspace{2cm}}.$$

· · · · · · · · · · · ·

$9;\ \frac{3}{2}$

$$\frac{6}{\frac{2}{3}} = 6 \times \frac{3}{2} = \overset{3}{6} \times \frac{3}{2}_1 = 9$$

134a.

Pieces of length $\frac{3}{4}$ are to be cut from 6 inches of tape. How many pieces of tape would result?

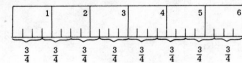

$$6 \div \frac{3}{4} = \underline{\hspace{2cm}} = 6 \times \underline{\hspace{2cm}}$$

· · · · · · · · · · · ·

$8; \dfrac{4}{3}$ $\dfrac{6}{3/4} = 6 \times \dfrac{4}{3} = 8$

---

135. How many doses of a drug can be dispensed if it is generally used in doses of $^6/_{100}$ grain for administration to infants and a total of 48 grains are available?

. . . .

$48 \div \dfrac{6}{100} = 48 \times \dfrac{100}{6} = 800$ doses   *48 grains must be subdivided into doses of $^6/_{100}$ grain each.*

135a.

How many $^3/_4$-grain doses are there in 9 grains?

. . . .

$9 \div \dfrac{3}{4} = 9 \times \dfrac{4}{3} = 12$

---

136. How many $^3/_4$-inch pieces can be cut from a 6-inch cord? The result should be (less than/greater than) 6, because _____

_____

_____.

. . . .

8; greater than   *There are 6 parts of length 1 inch in a 6-inch cord. The smaller the size of pieces cut off, the more pieces we can cut from the cord.*

$6 \div \dfrac{3}{4} = 6 \times \dfrac{4}{3} = 8$

---

137. $2 \div \dfrac{3}{4} =$ _____ ; $7 \div \dfrac{6}{5} =$ _____ .

. . . .

$\dfrac{8}{3}$ or $2^2/_3$; $\dfrac{35}{6}$ or $5^5/_6$

137a.

$12 \div \dfrac{3}{8} =$ _____ ; $\dfrac{4}{5} \div \dfrac{2}{9} =$ _____ .

. . . .

$32; \dfrac{18}{5}$ or $3\frac{3}{5}$

138. $2\frac{1}{10} \div \dfrac{63}{100} =$ _____ .

. . . .

$3\frac{1}{3}$ *Change $2\frac{1}{10}$ to an improper fraction; then follow the usual procedure for division:*

$$2\frac{1}{10} \div \frac{63}{100} = \frac{\overset{1}{\cancel{21}}}{\underset{1}{\cancel{10}}} \times \frac{\overset{10}{\cancel{100}}}{\underset{3}{\cancel{63}}} = \frac{10}{3} \text{ or } 3\frac{1}{3}$$

139. Digoxin is dispensed in a fruit-flavored syrup in doses of 0.05 ($\frac{5}{100}$) milligram. How many doses can be made if 6.1 ($6\frac{1}{10}$) milligrams are available?

. . . .

122

$$6\frac{1}{10} \div \frac{5}{100} = \frac{61}{10} \div \frac{5}{100} = \frac{61}{\underset{1}{\cancel{10}}} \times \frac{\overset{10}{\cancel{100}}}{5} =$$

122

139a.

How many bars of chocolate may be made from $7\frac{1}{4}$ ounces of chocolate if each bar weighs $1\frac{1}{2}$ ounce?

. . . .

$4\frac{5}{6}$, almost 5 bars of chocolate

$$7\frac{1}{4} \div 1\frac{1}{2} = \frac{29}{4} \div \frac{3}{2} = \frac{29}{\underset{2}{\cancel{4}}} \times \frac{\overset{1}{\cancel{2}}}{3} = \frac{29}{6} = 4\frac{5}{6}$$

140. How many $7\frac{1}{2}$-foot cars will fit into a space vacated by 17 9-foot cars?

. . . .

20 cars

Seventeen 9-foot cars occupy 153 feet.

$$153 \div 7\frac{1}{2} = 153 \div \frac{15}{2} = \overset{51}{\cancel{153}} \times \frac{2}{\cancel{15}_5} =$$

$$\frac{102}{5} = 20\frac{2}{5}$$

141. For each of the following problems indicate whether multiplication or division is necessary:

(a) Gantrisin is dispensed in doses of 15 grains. The doctor has ordered gantrisin for 5 different patients at 2 p.m. How many grains of gantrisin will be dispensed at 2 p.m.?

(b) If 15 grains of gantrisin are available and the doctor has prescribed doses of 5 grains each for a number of patients, how many doses can be administered?

. . . .

(a) multiplication (a) 1 patient gets 15 grains; 5 patients get 5 × 15 grains.

(b) division (b) 15 grains must be divided into doses of 5 grains each.

142. Complete the following table:

Problem	In this column write each problem as a product of fractions.	Use this column for final results.
$2\frac{3}{4} \times 4\frac{5}{6}$		
$6 \div \frac{2}{3}$		
$\frac{1}{300} \div \frac{1}{200}$		
$\frac{1}{16}$ $\frac{1}{24}$		

. . . .

Problem	In this column write each problem as a product of fractions.	Use this column for final results.
$2\frac{3}{4} \times 4\frac{5}{6}$	$\frac{11}{4} \times \frac{29}{6}$	$\frac{319}{24}$ or $13\frac{7}{24}$
$6 \div \frac{2}{3}$	$\frac{\overset{3}{\cancel{6}}}{1} \times \frac{3}{\underset{1}{\cancel{2}}}$	9
$\frac{1}{300} \div \frac{1}{200}$	$\frac{1}{\cancel{300}} \times \frac{\cancel{200}}{1}$	$\frac{2}{3}$
$\frac{1/16}{1/24}$	$\frac{1}{\underset{2}{\cancel{16}}} \times \frac{\overset{3}{\cancel{24}}}{1}$	$\frac{3}{2}$ or $1\frac{1}{2}$

143. Complete the following table:

Problem	In this column write each problem as a product of fractions.	Use this column for final results.
$\frac{1}{200} \div \frac{1}{10}$		
$\frac{1}{200} \div \frac{1}{100} \times 18$		
$\frac{1/20}{1/30} \times 15$		

. . . .

Problem	In this column write each problem as a product of fractions.	Use this column for final results.
$\dfrac{1}{200} \div \dfrac{1}{10}$	$\dfrac{1}{\cancel{200}_{20}} \times \dfrac{\cancel{10}^{1}}{1}$	$\dfrac{1}{20}$
$\dfrac{1}{200} \div \dfrac{1}{100} \times 18$	$\dfrac{1}{\cancel{200}_{2}} \times \dfrac{\cancel{100}^{1}}{1} \times \dfrac{\cancel{18}^{9}}{1}$	9
$\dfrac{1/20}{1/30} \times 15$	$\dfrac{1}{\cancel{20}_{2}} \times \dfrac{\cancel{30}^{3}}{1} \times \dfrac{15}{1}$	$\dfrac{45}{2}$ or $22\frac{1}{2}$

144. (a) The first step in the division of whole numbers or fractions by a fraction is to _____.

(b) If quantitative information q is provided about an item, and similar information s is provided about a subdivision of the item, how do you find the number of subdivisions into which an item has been divided?

. . . .

(a) See Item 4 in the Summary on the next page.

(b) See Item 6 in the Summary on the next page.

SUMMARY

1. To find the product of fractions, multiply the numerators and multiply the denominators.

   Example: $\dfrac{2}{3} \times \dfrac{7}{25} = \dfrac{14}{75}$

2. Simplify the process of multiplication by first dividing numerators and denominators by common divisors.

   Example: $\dfrac{\overset{1}{\cancel{2}}}{\underset{3}{\cancel{9}}} \times \dfrac{\overset{5}{\cancel{15}}}{\underset{4}{\cancel{8}}} = \dfrac{1 \times 5}{3 \times 4} = \dfrac{5}{12}$

3. To find the product of mixed numbers, change first to improper fractions.

   Example: $2\dfrac{3}{5} \times 7\dfrac{1}{2} = \dfrac{13}{\underset{1}{\cancel{5}}} \times \dfrac{\overset{3}{\cancel{15}}}{2} = \dfrac{39}{2} = 19\dfrac{1}{2}$

4. To divide a whole number or fraction by a second fraction, invert the *second* fraction and multiply.

   Example: $\dfrac{7}{9} \div \dfrac{2}{3} = \dfrac{7}{9} \times \dfrac{3}{2} = \dfrac{7}{6}$

5. If quantitative information q is given about one of n identical items, quantitative information about the n items may be found by multiplying q by n.

   Example: If the capacity of 1 of 10 identical glasses is 8 ounces, then the capacity of the 10 glasses is a total of $8 \times 10 = 80$ ounces.

6. If quantitative information q is provided for an item, and similar information s is provided for a subdivision of the item, divide q by s to find the number of subdivisions.

   Example: If $12\dfrac{1}{4}$ ounces of tuna are available for packaging into $3\dfrac{1}{2}$ ounce containers, how many such containers can be made?

   $12\dfrac{1}{4} \div 3\dfrac{1}{2} = \dfrac{49}{4} \div \dfrac{7}{2} = \dfrac{49}{4} \times \dfrac{2}{7} = \dfrac{14}{4} = \dfrac{7}{2} = 3\dfrac{1}{2}$

   Three containers can be made.

EXERCISES FOR EXTRA PRACTICE

1. Carry out the indicated operations.

(a) $\dfrac{2}{3} \times \dfrac{1}{4}$ (b) $\dfrac{7}{8} \times \dfrac{2}{3}$ (c) $\dfrac{3}{5} \times \dfrac{20}{9}$ (d) $7\dfrac{1}{2} \times \dfrac{1}{5}$

(e) $\dfrac{2}{5} \times 2\dfrac{1}{2}$ (f) $3\dfrac{3}{8} \times 21\dfrac{1}{3}$ (g) $5\dfrac{5}{6} \times 1\dfrac{11}{100}$ (h) $\dfrac{2}{3} \div \dfrac{6}{7}$

(i) $2\dfrac{1}{3} \div 5$ (j) $\dfrac{1}{2} \div \dfrac{3}{4}$ (k) $\dfrac{2}{3} \div \dfrac{4}{5}$ (l) $\dfrac{5}{6} \div \dfrac{8}{9}$

(m) $\dfrac{55}{1000} \div \dfrac{1}{25}$ (n) $3\dfrac{15}{7} \div 100$

. . . .

1. (a) $\dfrac{1}{6}$ (b) $\dfrac{7}{12}$ (c) $\dfrac{4}{3} = 1\dfrac{1}{3}$ (d) $\dfrac{3}{2} = 1\dfrac{1}{2}$

(e) 1   (f) 72   (g) $\dfrac{259}{40} = 6\dfrac{19}{40}$ (h) $\dfrac{7}{9}$

(i) $\dfrac{7}{15}$ (j) $\dfrac{2}{3}$ (k) $\dfrac{5}{6}$ (l) $\dfrac{15}{16}$

(m) $\dfrac{11}{8} = 1\dfrac{3}{8}$ (n) $\dfrac{9}{175}$

INVENTORY

Answer the following questions. If you have no errors, you are ready to advance to the next unit. Otherwise, study the relevant frames indicated on page 73. Then go back to the Proficiency Gauge on page 53.

1. Multiply $\dfrac{3}{7}$ by 4.

2. $\dfrac{3}{5} \times \dfrac{3}{7} = $ _____ .

3. $1\frac{1}{4} \times 2\frac{1}{3} = $ _____ .

4. $\dfrac{5}{9} \times \dfrac{3}{20} = $ _____ .

5. $\dfrac{14}{65} \times \dfrac{55}{21} = $ _____ .

6. $2\frac{1}{4} \times 1\frac{1}{15} = $ _____ .

7. Divide $\frac{4}{3}$ by $\frac{1}{3}$.

8. $\frac{5}{9} \div \frac{10}{21} =$ _____ .

9. $2\frac{2}{5} \div 2\frac{1}{4} =$ _____ .

10. How much fat content is in $3\frac{4}{5}$ pounds of hamburger if each pound contains $2\frac{1}{2}$ ounces of fat?

11. How many hamburgers may be made if each hamburger is to contain $4\frac{3}{8}$ ounces of meat and $62\frac{1}{2}$ ounces of meat are on hand?

. . . .

Answers

1. $\frac{12}{7}$ or $1\frac{5}{7}$ (Frames 106–110)

2. $\frac{9}{35}$ (Frames 111–121)

3. $\frac{35}{12}$ or $2\frac{11}{12}$ (Frames 121–122)

4. $\frac{1}{12}$ (Frames 119–121)

5. $\frac{22}{39}$ (Frames 119–121)

6. $\frac{12}{5}$ or $2\frac{2}{5}$ (Frames 119–123)

7. 4 (Frames 138–143)

8. $\frac{7}{6}$ or $1\frac{1}{6}$ (Frames 138–143)

9. $\frac{16}{15}$ or $1\frac{1}{15}$ (Frames 138–143)

10. $\frac{19}{2}$ or $9\frac{1}{2}$ ounces (Frames 123–126, 141)

11. $\frac{100}{7}$ or $14\frac{2}{7}$; this means 14 hamburgers and a little left over. (Frames 130, 133–136, 139–141)

RATIO AND PROPORTION

When two numbers of the same kind are compared by division, the result is called a ratio. In Alaska, the ratio of unmarried men to unmarried women is about 40 to 19, but in the District of Columbia this ratio is 41 to 42; in New York, the ratio is 15 to 14. The ratio of deaths from diseases of the heart to deaths from malignant neoplasms is about 5 to 2 in the United States.

A nurse must be able to calculate with ratios in preparing doses for oral administration. For instance, it may be necessary to dilute the stock solution of 1 to 1000 benzalkonium chloride in order to make a solution of 1 to 5000. The nurse may need to make up a potassium permanganate solution of 1 to 5000 from the crystals. Preparation of a child's dosage often requires that the nurse calculate the ratio of the child's weight to the weight of the average adult.

In this section, we discuss material that will enable the student to:

1. Know what is meant by "ratio," and express given information as a ratio using conventional notation.

2. Simplify ratios.

3. Judge the relative magnitude of two or more ratios.

4. Know what is meant by "proportion," "means," and "extremes," and write proportions from relevant data.

5. Solve a proportion with one unknown.

6. Apply the concept of ratio and proportion to the solution of simple verbal problems.

PROFICIENCY GAUGE

It is entirely possible that you do not need to review these topics. To gauge your proficiency, work out the following exercises. Uncover the printed answers only after you have answered all the questions. If you have no errors, skip ahead to Section 5.

1. It has been predicted that of approximately 60,000 girls who enter nursing school in a given year, about 20,000 withdraw. Find the ratio of students who withdraw to the total number of students who enter the nursing program.

2. The ratio of males to females in New York City is approximately 36:43. This means that of every 79 people, approximately how many are men?

3. Find the ratio of the value of 1 dime to the value of three quarters.

4. Simplify the following ratio: $\frac{1}{5}$:3.

5. Which ratio is greater, $\frac{1}{3}$:$\frac{1}{4}$ or 5:4?

6. Solve for x: 3:x = 1:40.

7. Find x in $\frac{x}{100} = \frac{50}{2500}$.

. . . .

Answers

1. $\frac{1}{3}$ or 1 : 3

2. 36

3. $\frac{2}{15}$ or 2 : 15

4. $\frac{1}{15}$ or 1 : 15

5. $\frac{1}{3}$: $\frac{1}{4}$

6. x = 120

7. 2

Read page 3 for instructions, if you have not already done so.

Writing a Ratio as a Common Fraction
Since there are two ways of expressing ratios, it is important to be able to convert from one to the other.

---

145. In Alaska, the ratio of unmarried men to unmarried women is about 40 to 19. This ratio may be expressed symbolically in two ways: $\frac{40}{19}$ or 40:19. Both symbols express the fact that for every 19 women there are _____ men.

. . . .

40

---

146. Use both types of symbols to express the ratio in the following statement: The ratio of doctors to nurses in the northeastern part of the United States is 1 to 2.

. . . .

$\frac{1}{2}$ or 1 : 2 $\dfrac{number\ of\ doctors}{number\ of\ nurses} = \dfrac{1}{2}$

---

147. From Frame 146, for every _____ doctor(s) in the northeastern United States there are _____ nurses.

. . . .

For every 1 doctor there are 2 nurses, for every 2 doctors, there are 4 nurses, etc.

---

148. Find the ratio of *nurses* to *doctors* in the northeastern United States.

. . . .

$\frac{2}{1}$ or 2 : 1 $\dfrac{number\ of\ nurses}{number\ of\ doctors} = \dfrac{2}{1}$

---

149. The ratio of deaths from diseases of the heart to deaths from malignant neoplasms is about 5 to 2 in the United States. Write this ratio symbolically in two ways.

. . . .

$\dfrac{5}{2}$, 5 : 2

$$\dfrac{number\ of\ deaths\ (heart)}{number\ of\ deaths\ (neoplasms)} = \dfrac{5}{2}$$

149a.

Write the ratio of deaths from malignant neoplasms to deaths from diseases of the heart in the United States

. . . .

2 : 5 or $\dfrac{2}{5}$

$$\dfrac{number\ of\ deaths\ (neoplasms)}{number\ of\ deaths\ (heart)} = \dfrac{2}{5}$$

---

150. Johnny weighs 30 pounds. The average adult weighs 150 pounds. What is the ratio of Johnny's weight to the weight of the average adult?

. . . .

30 : 150 or $\dfrac{30}{150}$ (may be reduced to $\frac{1}{5}$)

$$\dfrac{weight\ (Johnny)}{weight\ (average\ adult)} = \dfrac{30}{150}$$

150a.

Johnny's mother gives Johnny aspirin in 4 equal parts. What is the ratio of one of the small pieces to the whole aspirin? (Use both types of symbols.)

. . . .

$\dfrac{1}{4}$, 1 : 4

$$\dfrac{one\ part}{total\ number\ of\ parts} = \dfrac{1}{4}$$

---

151. If you answer 39 questions correctly on an examination that had 58 questions, what is the ratio of the number of correctly answered questions to the total number of questions?

. . . .

$\dfrac{39}{58}$ or 39 : 58

$$\dfrac{correct\ answers}{total\ number\ of\ questions} = \dfrac{39}{58}$$

---

152. Referring to the previous frame, what is the ratio of wrong answers to correct answers?

. . . .

$\dfrac{19}{39}$ or 19 : 39

$$\dfrac{\textit{number of wrong answers}}{\textit{number of correct answers}} = \dfrac{19}{39}$$

152a.

What is the ratio of wrong answers to the total number of answers?

. . . .

19 : 58

$$\dfrac{\textit{number of wrong answers}}{\textit{total number of answers}} = \dfrac{19}{58}$$

---

153. The ratio of a quantity A to a quantity B, measured in the same units, is nothing more than a common fraction, in which quantity _____ is the numerator and quantity _____ is the denominator.

. . . .

A is the numerator and B is
the denominator.

See page 98, Item 1.

---

154. The ratio of 1 to 3 is the common fraction _____ .

. . . .

$\dfrac{1}{3}$

154a.

The ratio 12 : 5, written as a common fraction, is _____ .

. . . .

$\dfrac{12}{5}$

---

155. The ratio x : 7, written as a common fraction, is _____ .

. . . .

$\dfrac{x}{7}$

155a.

The ratio $7 : x$, written as a common fraction, is _____ .

. . . .

$$\frac{7}{x}$$

156. The ratio of three pints to two quarts is nothing more than a common fraction, but the quantities must be measured in the same units. To compare pints with quarts, we must first change to comparable units. The number of pints in 2 quarts is _____, and therefore the ratio of 3 pints to 2 quarts if the ratio of 3 pints to _____ pints. In symbols, this is _____.

. . . .

The number of pints in 2 quarts is 4; thus, the ratio of 3 pints to 2 quarts is the same as the ratio of 3 pints to 4 pints or $\frac{3}{4}$ or 3:4.

157. Which one of the following comparisons could not be expressed by 1:3? (a) 1 dollar to 3 dollars, (b) 1 cent to 3 cents, (c) 1 pint to 3 pints, (d) 1 ounce to 3 pounds, (e) one inch to 3 inches.

. . . .

(d) $\dfrac{1 \ ounce}{3 \ pounds} = \dfrac{1 \ ounce}{48 \ ounces} = \dfrac{1}{48}, \ or \ 1:48, \ not \ \dfrac{1}{3}$

158. Which of the following comparisons would be expressed by 2:5? (a) 4 cents to 10 cents, (b) 2 cents to 5 dollars, (c) $\frac{2}{5}$, (d) There are 10 women for every 25 men.

. . . .

(a), (c), (d)   *(a), (c), and (d) all reduce to 2:5.*

(a) 4 cents to 10 cents is the same as 2 cents to 5 cents.

(b) This does not reduce to 2:5 because 2 cents to 5 dollars = 2 cents to 500 cents = 2:500.

(c) $\frac{2}{5}$ = 2:5.

(d) For every 10 women, there are 25 men; therefore, for every 2 women, there are 5 men.

159. Find the ratio of 1 nickel to 3 dollars (express in two ways).

. . . .

$\dfrac{1}{60}$ or 1 : 60 $\dfrac{1 \; nickel}{3 \; dollars} = \dfrac{5 \; cents}{300 \; cents} = \dfrac{1}{60}$ or 1 : 60

159a.

Find the ratio of 3 ounces to 2 pounds (assuming there are 16 ounces in 1 pound).

. . . .

$\dfrac{3}{32}$

160. The ratio 8 : 10 is nothing more than a common fraction with a numerator equal to _____ and a denominator equal to _____ . Write this ratio in common fraction form.

. . . .

$\dfrac{8}{10} = \dfrac{4}{5}$

160a.

The ratio 8 : 12 represents a common fraction with a numerator equal to _____ _____ and a denominator equal to _____ . Write this ratio in common fraction form.

. . . .

$\dfrac{8}{12} = \dfrac{2}{3}$

161. The ratio 40 : 25 represents a common fraction with a numerator equal to _____ _____ and a denominator equal to _____ . Write this ratio in common fraction form.

. . . .

$$\frac{40}{25} = \frac{8}{5}$$

161a.

The ratio $39 : 21$ represents a common fraction with a numerator equal to
_____ and a denominator equal to _____. Write this ratio in common fraction form.

. . . .

$$\frac{39}{21} = \frac{13}{7}$$

---

162. The ratio $3x : 15$ represents a common fraction with a numerator equal to
_____ and a denominator equal to _____. Write this ratio in common fraction form.

. . . .

$$\frac{3x}{15} = \frac{x}{5}$$

162a.

The ratio $6x : 15$ represents a common fraction with a numerator equal to
_____ and a denominator equal to _____. Write this ratio in common fraction form.

. . . .

$$\frac{6x}{15} = \frac{2x}{5}$$

---

163. The ratio $20 : 4x$ represents a common fraction with a numerator equal to
_____ and a denominator equal to _____. Write this ratio in common fraction form.

. . . .

$$\frac{20}{4x} = \frac{5}{x}$$

163a.

The ratio $15 : 6x$ represents a common fraction with a numerator equal to
_____ and a denominator equal to _____. Write this ratio in common fraction form.

. . . .

$$\frac{15}{6x} = \frac{5}{2x}$$

---

164. The ratio $12 : 20$ represents a common fraction with a numerator equal to
_____ and a denominator equal to _____. Write this ratio in common fraction form.

. . . .

$$\frac{12}{20} = \frac{3}{5}$$

---

165. In the ratio $12 : 20$, the first term is 12 and the second term is 20. In all ratios,
the first term is the _____ and the second term is the _____
_____ of the common fraction.

. . . .

first = numerator, second = denominator

---

166. Write the ratio $\frac{1}{2} : \frac{1}{3}$ as a common fraction and simplify.

. . . .

$\frac{3}{2}$ or $3 : 2$ $\frac{1}{2} : \frac{1}{3} = \frac{\frac{1}{2}}{\frac{1}{3}} = \frac{1}{2} \times \frac{3}{1} = \frac{3}{2}$

166a.

Write the ratio $\frac{1}{3} : \frac{3}{4}$ as a common fraction and simplify.

. . . .

$\frac{4}{9}$ $\frac{1}{3} : \frac{3}{4} = \frac{\frac{1}{3}}{\frac{3}{4}} = \frac{1}{3} \times \frac{4}{3} = \frac{4}{9}$

167. Write the ratio $\frac{x}{2} : \frac{1}{2}$ as a common fraction and simplify.

. . . .

x

$$\frac{x}{2} : \frac{1}{2} = \frac{x/2}{1/2} = \frac{x}{\cancel{2}} \times \frac{\cancel{2}}{1} = \frac{x}{1} = x$$

167a.

Write the ratio $\frac{2}{x} : \frac{3}{4}$ as a common fraction and simplify.

. . . .

$\frac{8}{3x}$

$$\frac{2}{x} : \frac{3}{4} = \frac{2}{x} \times \frac{4}{3} = \frac{8}{3x} \ \ or \ \ 8 : 3x$$

168. Write the ratio $5 : 6$ as a fraction. Write an equivalent ratio with a second term equal to 30. In your answer use both forms of ratio notation.

. . . .

$5 : 6 = \frac{5}{6} = \frac{25}{30}$ (multiplying the numerator and denominator by 5) $= 25 : 30$

168a.

Write the ratio $6 : 11$ as a fraction. Write an equivalent ratio with a second term equal to 33. In your answer use both forms.

. . . .

$6 : 11 = \frac{6}{11} = \frac{18}{33} = 18 : 33$

169. Write the ratio $7 : 9$ as a fraction. Write an equivalent ratio with a first term equal to 28. In your answer use both forms.

. . . .

$7 : 9 = \frac{7}{9} = \frac{28}{36} = 28 : 36$

169a.

Write the ratio 7 : 9 as a fraction. Write an equivalent ratio with a second term equal to 54. In your answer use both forms.

. . . .

$$7 : 9 = \frac{7}{9} = \frac{42}{54} = 42 : 54$$

---

170. The ratio of single men to single women is 7 : 6 in Ohio and 15 : 14 in New York. Where is a woman more likely to be able to find a husband?

. . . .

Ohio

In Ohio, there are 7 men for every 6 women; in New York there are 15 men for every 14 women. To compare the two ratios, the denominators must be the same. Use 42 as a least common denominator: 7 : 6 = 49 : 42 and 15 : 14 = 45 : 42. Therefore in Ohio there are 49 men for every 42 women but in New York there are only 45 men for every 42 women. The situation seems to be a little better for the women in Ohio.

170a.

A student correctly answered 12 out of 18 questions on her first test and 14 out of 20 questions on her second test. On which test did she get the better score?

. . . .

The second score was slightly better than the first.

$$\frac{12}{18} = \frac{2}{3}, \quad \frac{14}{20} = \frac{7}{10}$$

Change to equal denominators:

$$\frac{2}{3} = \frac{20}{30}, \quad \frac{7}{10} = \frac{21}{30}$$

$$\frac{21}{30} \text{ is better than } \frac{20}{30}$$

171. Brand *A* sells at the rate of 80 napkins for 12¢. Brand *B* sells the same quality napkins at the rate of 110 napkins for 16¢. Which is the better bargain?

. . . .

Brand *B*

There are 80 A napkins for every 12¢ or 20 for 3¢, since $^{80}/_{12} = ^{20}/_3$.

There are 110B napkins for every 16¢ or 55 for 8¢, since $^{110}/_{16} = ^{55}/_8$.

Now compare $^{20}/_3$ with $^{55}/_8$; change to equal denominators and compare $^{160}/_{24}$ with $^{165}/_{24}$.

There are 160 A napkins for 24¢ but 165 B napkins for 24¢.

172. Find the ratio of 3 inches to 2 feet.

. . . .

$\dfrac{1}{8}$ or 1 : 8

$\dfrac{3 \ inches}{2 \ feet} = \dfrac{3 \ inches}{24 \ inches} = \dfrac{1}{8}$

172a.

Find the ratio of 2 quarts to 3 gallons. (One gallon contains 4 quarts.)

. . . .

$\dfrac{1}{6}$ or 1 : 6

$\dfrac{2 \ quarts}{3 \ gallons} = \dfrac{2 \ quarts}{12 \ quarts} = \dfrac{1}{6}$

173. Complete the following sentence: In finding the ratio of 2 quantities it is important to express both quantities in _____ .

. . . .

See page 98, Item 2.

Simplifying Ratios

Carry out the indicated division and simplify the fraction.

---

174. To change the ratio $2\frac{1}{3} : 5$ to a simpler form without a mixed number, divide $2\frac{1}{3}$ by 5. Express the result as a ratio in 2 ways.

. . . .

$\frac{7}{15}$, 7:15

$2\frac{1}{3}:5 = \frac{7}{3} : 5 = \frac{7}{3} \div 5 = \frac{7}{3} \times \frac{1}{5} = \frac{7}{15}$

---

175. A nurse at Utopia Hospital gets 1 week of vacation for every 3 months that she works. Allowing $4\frac{1}{3}$ weeks in every month, what is the ratio of her vacation time to her working time?

. . . .

1 : 13

---

176. Which ratio is greater, $\frac{2}{3} : \frac{4}{5}$ or 6 : 7? Step 1: Change both ratios to common fractions. Step 2: Change the fractions to fractions that have the same _____. Solve the problem.

. . . .

6 : 7 is greater; denominator

$\frac{2}{3} : \frac{4}{5} = \frac{\frac{2}{3}}{\frac{4}{5}} = \frac{2}{3} \times \frac{5}{4} = \frac{5}{6}$

$6 : 7 = \frac{6}{7}$

Thus we are comparing $\frac{5}{6}$ with $\frac{6}{7}$.

Change $\frac{5}{6}$ and $\frac{6}{7}$ to fractions with like denominators:

$\frac{5}{6} = \frac{35}{42}$ *and* $\frac{6}{7} = \frac{36}{42}$

Since $\frac{36}{42}$ is greater than $\frac{35}{42}$, the ratio 6 : 7 is greater than $\frac{2}{3} : \frac{4}{5}$.

176a.

Which ratio is greater, $\frac{5}{6} : \frac{8}{9}$ or 31 : 32?

. . . .

31 : 32

$$\frac{5}{6} : \frac{8}{9} = \frac{\frac{5}{6}}{\frac{8}{9}} = \frac{5}{\underset{2}{6}} \times \frac{\overset{3}{9}}{8} = \frac{15}{16}$$

$$31 : 32 = \frac{31}{32}$$

$$But \; \frac{15}{16} = \frac{30}{32}$$

---

177. To simplify ratios, change them to what form?

. . . .

See page 98, Item 3.

Proportions

To understand and use the correct vocabulary, one must know the definitions of proportion, terms, means, and extremes. A simple method of solving proportions involves equating the product of the means with the product of the extremes.

---

178. A proportion is a mathematical statement that two ratios are equal, for example, $\frac{1}{2} = \frac{4}{8}$ or 1 : 2 = 4 : 8 (1 is to 2 as 4 is to 8). The terms of the ratios then become the _____ of the proportion.

. . . .

terms

---

179. Write the proportion stating the equality between the ratios ¾ and ⅝.

. . . .

$\frac{3}{4} = \frac{6}{8}$ or 3 : 4 = 6 : 8

180. The mathematical statement that $\frac{5}{9} = \frac{10}{18}$ is called a _____ .

. . . .

proportion

$\frac{5}{9}$ *is a ratio,* $\frac{10}{18}$ *is a ratio; the equation is called a proportion.*

---

181. Write a proportion using $\frac{7}{11}$.

. . . .

$\frac{7}{11} = \frac{14}{22}$ or $\frac{7}{11} = \frac{21}{33}$ or $\frac{7}{11} = \frac{28}{44}$, etc.

181a.

Write a proportion using $\frac{3}{8}$.

. . . .

$\frac{3}{8} = \frac{6}{16}$ or $\frac{3}{8} = \frac{24}{64}$, etc.

---

182. Write a proportion using $5 : 12$.

. . . .

$5 : 12 = 10 : 24$ or $5 : 12 = 20 : 48$, etc.

182a.

Write a proportion using $2 : 3$.

. . . .

$2 : 3 = 4 : 6$ or $2 : 3 = 8 : 12$, etc.

---

183. Consider the proportion $1 : 3 = 2 : 6$. Which numbers, on both sides, are at the extreme ends of the equation?

. . . .

1, 6

183a.

Consider the proportion $3:8 = 12:32$. Which numbers, on both sides, are at the extreme ends of the equation?

. . . .

3, 32

184. The numbers, on both sides, at the *extreme* ends of the equation written in 183 are called the _____ .

. . . .

extremes (what originality!)

185. Consider the proportion $7:5 = 21:15$. Which numbers are the extremes?

. . . .

7, 15

185a.

Consider the proportion $1:2 = 4:8$. Which numbers are the extremes?

. . . .

1, 8

186. Consider the proportion $\frac{3}{4} = \frac{6}{8}$. Which numbers are the extremes?

. . . .

3, 8   *Note that* $\dfrac{3}{4} = \dfrac{6}{8}$ *is equivalent to* $3:4 = 6:8$.

186a.

Consider the proportion $\frac{6}{8} = \frac{3}{4}$. Which numbers are the extremes?

. . . .

6, 4   *Note that $\dfrac{6}{8} = \dfrac{3}{4}$ is equivalent to 6 : 8 = 3 : 4.*

---

187. In the proportions 8 : 2 = 4 : 1, which numbers are the means?

. . . .

2, 4   *The numbers 8 and 1 are the extremes; the numbers 2 and 4 are the means.*

187a.

In the proportion 7 : 5 = 21 : 15, which numbers are the means?

. . . .

5, 21   *7 and 15 are the extremes; 5 and 21 are the means.*

---

188. In the proportion $^{10}\!/_{34} = {}^{5}\!/_{17}$, which numbers are the means?

. . . .

34, 5   *Since $\dfrac{10}{34} = \dfrac{5}{17}$ is equivalent to 10 : 34 = 5 : 17, 34 and 5 are the means.*

188a.

In the proportion $^{5}\!/_{2} = {}^{15}\!/_{6}$, which numbers are the means?

. . . .

2, 15   *Since $\dfrac{5}{2} = \dfrac{15}{6}$ is equivalent to 5 : 2 = 15 : 6, 2 and 15 are the means.*

---

189. Define proportion.

. . . .

Check with page 98 Item 4.

190. Find the product of (multiply) the extremes in the proportion $2:3 = 10:15$; also find the product of (multiply) the means.

. . . .

30; 30   *2 × 15 = 30; 3 × 10 = 30*

190a.

Given the proportion $6:8 = 3:4$, find the product of the means. Find the product of the extremes.

. . . .

8 × 3 = 24; 6 × 4 = 24

191. Given the proportion $\frac{5}{8} = \frac{20}{32}$, find the product of the means and the product of the extremes.

. . . .

160; 160   *The product of the means is 8 × 20 = 160; the product of the extremes is 5 × 32 = 160.*

191a.

Given the proportion $\frac{2}{5} = \frac{6}{15}$, find the product of the means and the product of the extremes.

. . . .

30; 30   *The product of the means is 5 × 6 = 30; the product of the extremes is 2 × 15 = 30.*

192. In any true proportion, the product of the means is (always equal to/sometimes equal to/never equal to) the product of the extremes.

. . . .

always equal to   *See page 98, Item 5.*

193. If the product of the means does not equal the product of the extremes, what can be said about two ratios?

. . . .

They are not equal, or the proportion is not true.

___

194. Is this proportion true? $1:2 = 2:3$. Explain how you know. Test by finding the product of the means and the product of the extremes.

. . . .

No.

The product of the means is 4; the product of the extremes is 3. In a true proportion, the product of the means must equal the product of the extremes.

___

194a.

Which, if any, of the following are true proportions? (a) $15:6 = 8:3$

(b) $\dfrac{3}{12} = \dfrac{25}{10}$ (c) $\dfrac{1}{50}:1 = \dfrac{1}{25}:2$ (d) $\dfrac{1/2}{2} = \dfrac{100}{50}$

. . . .

(c)

(a) $15:6 = 8:3$ is not a true proportion because $15 \times 3 = 45$ but $6 \times 8 = 48$.

(b) $\dfrac{3}{12} = \dfrac{25}{10}$ is not a true proportion because $3 \times 10 = 30$ but $12 \times 25 = 300$.

(c) $\dfrac{1}{50}:1 = \dfrac{1}{25}:2$ is a true proportion because $\dfrac{1}{\underset{25}{50}} \times {}_1\cancel{2} = \dfrac{1}{25}$ and $1 \times \dfrac{1}{25} = \dfrac{1}{25}$.

(d) $\dfrac{1/2}{2} = \dfrac{100}{50}$ is not a true proportion because $\dfrac{1}{2} \times 50 = 25$ but $2 \times 100 = 200$.

195. Given the proportion $x/6 = 15/9$, find the product of the means and the product of the extremes.

. . . .

90; $9x$

To find the product of the means, multiply 6 X 15. Result: 90. To find the product of the extremes, multiply 9 X x. Result: 9x.

195a.

Given the proportion $x/3 = 160/24$, find the product of the means and the product of the extremes.

. . . .

480; $24x$

3 X 160 = 480 (product of means); 24 X x = 24x (product of extremes)

---

196. Given the proportion $7/x = 21/15$, find the product of the means and the product of the extremes.

. . . .

$21x$; 105

21 X x = 21x; 7 X 15 = 105

196a.

Given the proportion $2/3 \times x/15$, find the product of the means and the product of the extremes.

. . . .

$3x$; 30

---

197. Refer to Frame 195. If $x/6 = 15/9$ is a true proportion, then 90 is (greater than/equal to/less than) $9x$. Explain how you know.

. . . .

equal to

90 is the product of the means; 9x is the product of the extremes. In a true proportion, the product of the means equals the product of the extremes.

198. The value of $2x$ must be _____ , if the following is to be a true proportion: $\frac{2}{10} = \frac{5}{x}$.

. . . .

50

The product of the extremes ($2x$) is equal to the product of the means (50).

198a.

Find the value of $7x$ that will make the following a true proportion: $\frac{150}{x} = \frac{7}{10}$.

. . . .

1500

$7x = 150 \times 10 = 1500$

---

199. Find the product of the means and the product of the extremes. Then find x if the following is to be a true proportion: $\frac{7}{15} = \frac{2}{x}$.

. . . .

$\frac{30}{7}$ or $4\frac{2}{7}$

The product of the means (30) must equal the product of the extremes ($7x$).

$7x = 30$

Divide both sides of the equation by 7:

$\frac{\cancel{7}x}{\cancel{7}} = \frac{30}{7}$

$x = \frac{30}{7} = 4\frac{2}{7}$

199a.

Find x if the following is to be true: $\frac{8}{25} = \frac{7}{x}$.

. . . .

$\frac{175}{8}$ or $21\frac{7}{8}$

The product of the means (175) must equal the product of the extremes ($8x$).

$8x = 175$

Divide both sides of the equation by 8:

$\frac{8x}{8} = \frac{175}{8}$

$x = 21\frac{7}{8}$

200. If, in a certain proportion, the product of the means = $\frac{5}{2}x$ and the product of the extremes = 15, what value would x have in order that the proportion be true?

. . . .

$x = 6$

Since the product of the means equals the product of the extremes, $\frac{5}{2}x = 15.$

Divide both sides by $\frac{5}{2}$ *(or multiply by* $\frac{2}{5}$ *):*

$$\frac{\cancel{2}}{\cancel{5}} \times \frac{\cancel{5}}{\cancel{2}}x = \frac{2}{\cancel{5}_1} \times \cancel{15}^3 = 6$$

200a.

From a certain proportion, the product of the means is $\frac{4x}{7}$ and the product of the extremes is 200. Find x to make the proportion true.

. . . .

$x = 350$

$$\frac{4x}{7} = 200$$

Divide both sides by $\frac{4}{7}$ *(multiply by* $\frac{7}{4}$ *):*

$$\frac{\cancel{7}}{\cancel{4}} \times \frac{\cancel{4}}{\cancel{7}}x = \frac{7}{\cancel{4}} \times \cancel{200}^{50} = 350$$

---

201. Find the products of means and extremes and solve for x: $2:x = \frac{5}{100}:100.$

. . . .

$x = 4000$

$$\frac{5}{100}x = 200$$

$$or \ \frac{1}{20}x = 200$$

$$20 \times \frac{1}{20}x = 20 \times 200$$

$$x = 4000$$

202. Find x if $\frac{4}{5} : 3 = x : 6$.

. . . .

$\frac{8}{5}$ or $1\frac{3}{5}$

$3x = \frac{24}{5}$

Divide both sides by 3 (multiply by $\frac{1}{3}$):

$3x \times \frac{1}{3} = \frac{24}{5} \times \frac{1}{3}$

$\frac{3x}{3} = \frac{8}{5}$

$x = \frac{8}{5}$ *or* $1\frac{3}{5}$

---

203. To solve a proportion, solve the equation produced by setting _____
     equal to _____ .

. . . .

Check with page 98, Item 6.

SUMMARY

1. The ratio of x to y may be written in ratio notation, $x:y$, or as a common fraction, $\frac{x}{y}$.

   Example: $3:4 = \frac{3}{4}$

2. In finding the ratio of two quantities, both quantities should be expressed in the same units.

   Example: Two lengths may be compared as follows: 5 inches : 2 feet = 5 inches : 24 inches = 5 : 24 or $\frac{5}{24}$.

3. To simplify ratios, carry out the indicated division and simplify the fraction.

   Example: $15:6 = \frac{15}{6} = \frac{5}{2}$ or $5:2$

4. A proportion is a mathematical statement that two ratios are equal.

   Example: $15:6 = 5:2$ or $\frac{15}{6} = \frac{5}{2}$

5. In a proportion, the product of the means is equal to the product of the extremes.

   Example: If $15:6 = 5:2$, then $6 \times 5 = 15 \times 2$.

6. To solve a proportion, write the equation produced by setting the product of the means equal to the product of the extremes.

   Example: If $\frac{x}{2} = \frac{7}{15}$, then $15x = 14$ and $x = \frac{14}{15}$.

EXERCISES FOR EXTRA PRACTICE

1. Find the following ratios in simplest form.

   (a) 1 day to 1 week   (b) 1 month to 1 year   (c) 3 feet to 2 yards

   (d) 9 inches to 3 feet   (e) $\frac{1}{2}$ pound to 5 ounces   (f) 3 quarters to 7 dimes

2. Solve the following proportions.

   (a) $\frac{x}{100} = \frac{33}{10}$ (b) $\frac{x}{30} = \frac{60}{100}$ (c) $\frac{x}{2000} = \frac{15}{100}$

   (d) $\frac{20}{100} = \frac{x}{8}$ (e) $\frac{2}{y} = \frac{25}{100}$ (f) $\frac{16}{5} = \frac{5}{y}$

   (g) $\frac{4}{y} = \frac{15}{100}$ (h) $\frac{3}{4} = \frac{x}{100}$ (i) $\frac{8}{13} = \frac{100}{x}$

. . . .

Answers

1. (a) $\frac{1}{7}$ (b) $\frac{1}{12}$ (c) $\frac{3}{6} = \frac{1}{2}$

   (d) $\frac{9}{36} = \frac{1}{4}$ (e) $\frac{8}{5}$ (f) $\frac{75}{70} = \frac{15}{14}$

2. (a) 330   (b) 18   (c) 300

   (d) $\frac{8}{5}$ (e) 8   (f) $\frac{25}{16}$

   (g) $\frac{80}{3}$ (h) 75   (i) $\frac{325}{2}$

INVENTORY

Answer the following questions. If you have everything right, you are ready to advance to the next section. If you have some errors, study the relevant frames indicated. Then work out the Proficiency Gauge on page 75.

1. In a study of 600 student nurses, it was found that 250 students had de-cided on a nursing career early, that is, before the age of 14. What is the ratio of students who had made early career decisions to the total student population?

2. Among second year students studying nursing, the ratio of those satisfied with the curriculum to those who are dissatisfied is about 37 : 14. This means that of every 51 nursing students, approximately how many are likely to be satisfied with the curriculum?

3. Simplify the ratio $\frac{1}{3}$: 5.

4. Find the ratio of 3 inches to 2 yards.

5. Which ratio is greater, $\frac{1}{5}$: $\frac{1}{4}$ or 3 : 4?

6. Solve for x if 5 : 100 = x : 2000.

7. Find x if $^{250}/_x = ^5/_{20}$.

. . . .

Answers

Compare your answers with the correct answers below. If you have no errors, advance to Section 5. Otherwise study the relevant frames and then work out the Proficiency Gauge on page 75.

1. 5 : 12 or $\frac{5}{12}$ (Frames 145—152)

2. 37 (Frames 145—146)

3. 1 : 15 or $\frac{1}{15}$ (Frames 160—167, 174—177)

4. 1 : 24 or $\frac{1}{24}$ (Frames 156—159)

5. $\frac{1}{5}$: $\frac{1}{4}$ is greater (Frames 170—172, 176)

6. x = 100 (Frames 195—202)

7. x = 1000 (Frames 168—169)

PERCENT

Percent is indispensable because it provides one of the most efficient ways of comparing quantities. Consider how often the symbol is used.

The distribution of intelligence among people is roughly as follows: 22½% inferior, 55% average, 22½% superior. Of all lung tumors, 72% develop between the ages of 40 and 72 years. Only 70% of ingested phosphorus is absorbed by the body. The head of a human is 25% of its total length in infancy and only 11% of its total length in adulthood.

The nurse must be able to determine, for example, the gastric acidity of a patient after gastric surgery, knowing that normal acidity after histamine is 25% to 50%. He or she may be instructed to cocainize a patient's eye with a 4% or 5% solution of cocaine. One may need to calculate the percent strength of a 10-ounce solution containing 2 drams of drug. Sometimes we must know how many minims of a 0.1% solution to use in administering 1/100 grain of atropine sulfate.

In this section, we discuss the concept of percent so that the student is able to:

1. Change any number from percent form to mixed number form, or the reverse.

2. Find any percent of a given number.

PROFICIENCY GAUGE

Work out the following exercises. Uncover the printed answers at the bottom of this page only after you have answered all the questions.

1. Change to common fractions or mixed numbers: 23%, $1\frac{2}{3}$%, $\frac{1}{10}$%, 203%, $\frac{1}{2}$%.

2. A bank gives $5\frac{1}{4}$% interest at the end of each calendar year on all balances that are at least one year old. If your balance at the beginning of the year had been $2800, how much interest should you receive?

3. Change to percent: $\frac{312}{1000}$, $\frac{1}{6}$, $1\frac{4}{5}$, 38.

4. An evening gown is reduced from $60 to $55. What percent reduction is this?

5. All but 10% of the available funds have been used. What percent has been used?

6. What percent of 15 is 25?

. . . .

Answers

1. $23\% = \frac{23}{100}$, $1\frac{2}{3}\% = \frac{1}{60}$, $\frac{1}{10}\% = \frac{1}{1000}$, $203\% = 2\frac{3}{100}$, $\frac{1}{2}\% = \frac{1}{200}$

2. $147

3. $\frac{312}{1000} = 31\frac{1}{5}\%$; $\frac{1}{6} = 16\frac{2}{3}\%$; $1\frac{4}{5}\% = 180\%$; $38 = 3800\%$

4. $8\frac{1}{3}\%$

5. 90%

6. $166\frac{2}{3}\%$

If you have errors, go on to Frame 204. Otherwise skip ahead to Section 6.

Read page 3 for instructions, if you have not already done so.

Meaning of Percent

Percents are just ratios with the denominator 100. Since these ratios are particularly convenient, they have their own special symbols.

---

204. In every group of 100 people in the United States, we are likely to find 22 people with above-average intelligence. Find the ratio of people with above-average intelligence to the total population.

. . . .

$22 : 100$ or $\dfrac{22}{100}$

204a.

In every group of 100 married women, we are likely to find 41 working wives. What is the ratio of working wives to the total number of married women?

. . . .

$41 : 100$ or $\dfrac{41}{100}$

---

205. The ratio of people with above-average intelligence to the total population is $\frac{22}{100}$; more simply, 22% (twenty-two percent) of the population has above-average intelligence. The symbol $\frac{22}{100}$, has been replaced by _____ .

. . . .

22%

205a.

The ratio of working wives to the total number of married women is $\frac{41}{100}$; more simply, 41% of married women work. The symbol $\frac{41}{100}$ has been replaced by _____ .

. . . .

41%

---

206. The ratio of married women to all women workers is 63/100; more simply,
_____ of women workers are married. (What percent?)

. . . .

63%

206a.

The ratio of park land to all land in New York City is $^{17}/_{100}$; more simply,
_____ of New York City land is park land.

. . . .

17%

---

207. About 25% of nursing students decide upon their careers before they are 10
years old. The ratio of these students to all nursing students is _____ .

. . . .

$\frac{25}{100}, \frac{1}{4}$, 25 : 100, or 1 : 4

207a.

About 10% of nursing students decide upon their careers after the age of 17.
The ratio of these students to all nursing students is _____ .

. . . .

$\frac{10}{100}, \frac{1}{10}$, 10 : 100, or 1 : 10

---

208. 25% is equivalent to $^{25}/_{100}$. The % sign replaces part of $^{25}/_{100}$. Circle the part of
$^{25}/_{100}$ that is replaced by "%."

. . . .

$\left(\!/100\right)$, that is, "%" symbolizes division by 100.

208a.

17% is equivalent to $^{17}/_{100}$. The % sign replaces part of $^{17}/_{100}$. Circle the part of $^{17}/_{100}$ replaced by "%."

. . . .

209. 5 % is equivalent to $^{5}/_{100}$. 12% is equivalent to _____ . 27% is equivalent to _____ .

. . . .

$12\% = \dfrac{3}{25}$ $12\% = \dfrac{12}{100}, \dfrac{3}{25}, \text{ or } 3 : 25$

$27\% = \dfrac{27}{100}$ $27\% = \dfrac{27}{100}, \text{ or } 27 : 100$

209a.

33% is equivalent to _____ .

. . . .

$\dfrac{33}{100}$ or 33 : 100

Changing Percents to Common Fractions
Wherever "%" is seen, division by 100 may be substituted.

210. The word "percent" comes from the Latin, *per centum*, meaning "by the hundred," "in a hundred," "per hundred," or "divided by 100." The symbol %, containing a slant line and two zeros, has the symbols that are found in 100. Change 80% to a common fraction.

. . . .

$80\% = \dfrac{80}{100}$ or $\dfrac{4}{5}$

211. In the following paragraph, wherever you see a number expressed in percent form, change it to a common fraction:

The increase in the number of working wives from 1960 to 1970 accounted for 72% of the gain in the total number of women workers. The proportion of married women who work jumped from 32% in 1960 to 41% in 1970. In 1970, working wives constituted 65% of all women workers as compared with 55% in 1960.

. . . .

$72\% = \dfrac{72}{100} = \dfrac{18}{25}$; $32\% = \dfrac{32}{100} = \dfrac{8}{25}$; $41\% = \dfrac{41}{100}$;

$65\% = \dfrac{65}{100} = \dfrac{13}{20}$; $55\% = \dfrac{55}{100} = \dfrac{11}{20}$

---

212. Just after World War II, the cost of living went up 150%. Write this percent in fractional form and simplify.

. . . .

$\dfrac{150}{100} = \dfrac{3}{2}$

212a.

Bread is 395% more expensive than it was before World War II. In fractional form this is _____ .

. . . .

$\dfrac{395}{100} = 3\,^{95}\!/_{100}$ or $3\,^{19}\!/_{20}$

---

213. Express without a percent sign and simplify ½%.

. . . .

$\dfrac{1}{200}$ $\dfrac{½}{100} = \dfrac{1}{2} \times \dfrac{1}{100} = \dfrac{1}{200}$

214. Express each of the following without a percent sign and simplify: (a) $\frac{3}{4}$%

(b) 75%

. . . .

(a) $\frac{3}{400}$

(b) $\frac{3}{4}$

(a) $\frac{3}{4}\% = \frac{3}{4} \div 100$

$= \frac{3}{4} \times \frac{1}{100}$

$= \frac{3}{400}$

(b) $75\% = 75 \div 100$

$= 75 \times \frac{1}{100}$

$= \frac{3}{4}$

214a.

Express each of the following without a % sign and simplify: (a) $\frac{1}{4}$%   (b) 25%

. . . .

(a) $\frac{1}{4}\% = \frac{1}{400}$

(b) $25\% = \frac{1}{4}$

(a) $\frac{1}{4}\% = \frac{\frac{1}{4}}{100} = \frac{1}{400}$

(b) $25\% = \frac{25}{100} = \frac{1}{4}$

---

215. (a) Change $2\frac{1}{7}$ to a fraction.   (b) Change $2\frac{1}{7}$% to a fraction and simplify.

. . . .

(a) $2\frac{1}{7} = \frac{15}{7}$

(b) $2\frac{1}{7} = \frac{3}{140}$

$2\frac{1}{7}\% = \frac{15}{7}\% = \frac{\frac{15}{7}}{100} = \frac{15}{700} = \frac{3}{140}$

215a.

(a) Change $3\frac{1}{5}$ to a fraction.   (b) Change $3\frac{1}{5}$% to a fraction and simplify.

. . . .

(a) $3\frac{1}{5} = \frac{16}{5}$

(b) $3\frac{1}{5}\% = \frac{4}{125}$ $3\frac{1}{5}\% = \frac{16}{5}\% = \frac{16/5}{100} = \frac{16}{500} = \frac{4}{125}$

---

216. What does "%" mean?

. . . .

Check page 123, Item 1.

---

217. Complete the following table (simplify all fractions):

Percent	Fraction, Mixed Number, or Whole Number
2%	$\frac{2}{100} = \frac{1}{50}$
123%	$\frac{123}{100} = 1\,^{23}/_{100}$
$2\frac{1}{2}\%$	
$\frac{7}{10}\%$	
425%	
100%	
25%	
200%	

. . . .

$2\frac{1}{2}\% = \frac{5}{2}\% = \frac{5/2}{100} = \frac{5}{2} \times \frac{1}{100} = \frac{5}{200} = \frac{1}{40}$

$\frac{7}{10}\% = \frac{7/10}{100} = \frac{7}{10} \times \frac{1}{100} = \frac{7}{1000}$

$425\% = \frac{425}{100} = 4\frac{25}{100} = 4\frac{1}{4}$

$100\% = \frac{100}{100} = 1$

$25\% = \frac{25}{100} = \frac{1}{4}$

$200\% = \frac{200}{100} = 2$

218. If you heard that 20% of your class, in which there are 65 students, failed the final examination, how many students would you know had failed?

. . . .

13 $20\% = \dfrac{20}{100} = \dfrac{1}{5}, \dfrac{1}{5} \times 65 = 13$

219. If 20% of the students failed, _____% passed.

. . . .

80%

220. If 16% of a loaf of bread had been nibbled away by mice, what percentage of the loaf remained?

. . . .

84%   One loaf = 100%; therefore 84% of the loaf remained.

221. In a certain nursing class 15% of the students married doctors. What percentage did not marry doctors? If there were 120 in the class, how many married doctors?

. . . .

85%; 18   The total number of students is 100% of the class. If 15% married doctors, 85% did not. In the class of 120, 15% of the class is 18 students since

$$15\% \times 120 = \dfrac{\cancel{15}^{3}}{\cancel{100}_{5}} \times \cancel{120}^{6} = 18.$$

221a.

About 44% of nursing students plan to work in a nursing specialty. What percentage do not plan to work in a specialty? About how many in a class of 300 expect to work in a specialty?

. . . .

56%; 132 $100\% - 44\% = 56\%$

$$44\% \times 300 = \frac{44}{100} \times 300 = 132$$

---

222. Students are improving all the time. On a certain exam, the average grade used to be 60. Now students get 12% more on the average than 60. How many points higher is the average grade now? What is the average grade now?

. . . .

$\frac{12}{100} \times 60 = 7\frac{1}{5}$ points higher; $60 + 7\frac{1}{5} = 67\frac{1}{5}$, new average grade

---

223. If a man loses 13% of his inheritance (amounting to $5270) in the stock market, what percentage remained and what did it amount to?

. . . .

87%; $4584.90   *(by multiplying 5270 $\times$ .87)*

---

224. A solution containing 48 ounces of water lost 20% of the water because of evaporation. How many ounces of water are left?

. . . .

$38\frac{2}{5}$ *The original solution had 100% (all) of its required amount of water. Having lost 20% of the water, 80% was left.*

80% of $48 = \frac{80}{100} \times 48 = \frac{4}{5} \times 48 = \frac{192}{5} =$

$38\frac{2}{5}$ ounces

---

225. In one year, the price of vitamins has gone up by 10%. If a capsule used to cost 3 cents, how much does it now cost? How much do 100 capsules cost?

. . . .

$3\frac{3}{10}$ cents; $3.30   *$10\%$ of $3 = 10\% \times 3 = \frac{1}{10} \times 3 = \frac{3}{10}$*

(amount of increase)

$3 + \frac{3}{10} = \frac{33}{10}$ cents (present cost)

100 capsules cost $\frac{33}{10} \times 100 = \frac{33}{\cancel{10}_1} \times \cancel{100}^{10}$
$= 330$ cents $= \$3.30$

226. How many ounces of glycerin are there in 30 ounces of a 60% solution of glycerin?

. . . .

18

Replace 60% by $\dfrac{60}{100}$.

$\dfrac{\text{number of ounces of glycerin}}{\text{number of ounces of solution}} = \dfrac{x}{30} = \dfrac{60}{100}$

$x = \dfrac{60}{100} \times 30$

$\quad = \dfrac{6}{10} \times 30$

$\quad = 6 \times 3 = 18$

---

227. How many ounces of sodium biphosphate are present in 8 ounces of a 20% solution of sodium biphosphate?

. . . .

1³⁄₅

$\dfrac{\text{number of ounces of sodium biphosphate}}{\text{number of ounces of solution}} =$

$\dfrac{x}{8} = \dfrac{20}{100}$

$x = \dfrac{20}{100} \times 8$

$\quad = \dfrac{1}{5} \times 8$

$\quad = \dfrac{8}{5}$ *or* $1^{3}\!/_{5}$

---

228. To find $x\%$ of a number, what steps do you follow?

. . . .

Check page 123, Item 2.

Changing Common Fractions to Percents

Use proportions to obtain percents.

---

229. Your boyfriend or girlfriend has just given you a watch with an 18-carat gold wristband. This is almost pure gold, but not entirely. What percentage of pure gold is the band? (24 carats would be pure gold.)

. . . .

75%

$$\frac{18}{24} = x\%$$

$$\frac{18}{24} = \frac{x}{100}$$

$$\frac{3}{4} = \frac{x}{100}$$

*This is solved easily by the fundamental principle of fractions. Since 100 is 25 ×
4, x is 25 × 3 and $\frac{18}{24}$ = 75%.*

---

230. A 6-carat band would be what percentage of pure gold?

. . . .

25%

$$\frac{6}{24} = x\%$$

$$\frac{1}{4} = \frac{x}{100}$$

*Since 100 is 25 × 4, x is 25 × 1 = 25 and
$\frac{6}{24}$ is 25%.*

---

231. Change to percents: (a) 1   (b) $\frac{1}{2}$ (c) $\frac{1}{4}$ (d) $\frac{2}{5}$

. . . .

(a) 100%

(b) 50%

(c) 25%

(d) 40%

(a) $1 = x\%$

$1 = \dfrac{x}{100}$

$100 = x$

$1 = 100\%$

(b) $\dfrac{1}{2} = x\%$

$\dfrac{1}{2} = \dfrac{x}{100}$

$x = 50$

$\dfrac{1}{2} = 50\%$

(c) $\dfrac{1}{4} = x\%$

$\dfrac{1}{4} = \dfrac{x}{100}$

$x = 25$

$\dfrac{1}{4} = 25\%$

(d) $\dfrac{2}{5} = x\%$

$\dfrac{2}{5} = \dfrac{x}{100}$

$x = 40$

$\dfrac{2}{5} = 40\%$

231a.

Change to percents: (a) $\dfrac{3}{10}$ (b) $\dfrac{7}{20}$ (c) $\dfrac{9}{25}$ (d) $\dfrac{11}{50}$

. . . .

(a) $\dfrac{3}{10} = 30\%$

(b) $\dfrac{7}{20} = 35\%$

(c) $\dfrac{9}{25} = 36\%$

(d) $\dfrac{11}{50} = 22\%$

(a) $\dfrac{3}{10} = x\%$

$\dfrac{3}{10} = \dfrac{x}{100}$

$x = 30$

$\dfrac{3}{10} = 30\%$

(b) $\dfrac{7}{20} = x\%$

$\dfrac{7}{20} = \dfrac{x}{100}$

$x = 35$

$\dfrac{7}{20} = 35\%$

(c) $\dfrac{9}{25} = x\%$

$\dfrac{9}{25} = \dfrac{x}{100}$

$x = 36$

$\dfrac{9}{25} = 36\%$

(d) $\dfrac{11}{50} = x\%$

$\dfrac{11}{50} = \dfrac{x}{100}$

$x = 22$

$\dfrac{11}{50} = 22\%$

---

232. Express $\frac{1}{8}$ as a percent.

. . . .

$12\frac{1}{2}\%$

$$\frac{1}{8} = x\%$$

$$\frac{1}{8} = \frac{x}{100}$$

$$8x = 100$$

$$x = 12\frac{1}{2}$$

$$\frac{1}{8} = 12\frac{1}{2}\%$$

232a.

Express $\frac{3}{7}$ as a percent.

. . . .

$42\frac{6}{7}\%$

$$\frac{3}{7} = x\%$$

$$\frac{3}{7} = \frac{x}{100}$$

$$7x = 300$$

$$x = 42\frac{6}{7}$$

$$\frac{3}{7} = 42\frac{6}{7}\%$$

233. Express $1\frac{5}{8}$ as a percent.

. . . .

$162\frac{1}{2}\%$

$$1\frac{5}{8} = x\%$$

$$\frac{13}{8} = \frac{x}{100}$$

$$8x = 1300$$

$$x = 162\frac{1}{2}$$

$$1\frac{5}{8} = 162\frac{1}{2}\%$$

233a.

Express $11\frac{2}{3}$ as a percent.

. . . .

$1166\frac{2}{3}\%$

$11\frac{2}{3} = x\%$

$\dfrac{35}{3} = \dfrac{x}{100}$

$3x = 3500$

$x = 1166\frac{2}{3}$

$11\frac{2}{3} = 1166\frac{2}{3}\%$

---

234. Express 250 as a percent.

. . . .

25,000%

$250 = x\%$

$250 = \dfrac{x}{100}$

$x = 25,000$

234a.

Express 12 as a percent.

. . . .

1200%

$12 = x\%$

$12 = \dfrac{x}{100}$

$x = 1200$

---

235. Correct the error in the following statement: $450 = 4\frac{1}{2}\%$.

. . . .

You could say $450 = 45,000\%$, not $4\frac{1}{2}\%$; or $4\frac{1}{2}\% = \dfrac{9}{2}\%$ or $\dfrac{9}{200}$, not 450

236. If a person with an average daily total consumption of 3000 calories has about 450 calories for breakfast, what percentage of his total daily intake is consumed at breakfast?

. . . .

15%

$$\frac{450}{3000} = x\%$$

$$\frac{450}{3000} = \frac{x}{100}$$

$$\frac{15}{100} = \frac{x}{100}$$

$$x = 15$$

237. If, on a National League for Nurses Achievement Examination in Pharmacology containing 130 questions, you answer 75 correctly, what should your score be, given as a percent?

. . . .

58%

$$\frac{75}{130} = x\%$$

$$\frac{\overset{15}{\cancel{75}}}{\underset{26}{\cancel{130}}} = \frac{x}{100}$$

$$26x = 1500$$

$$x = 57\tfrac{18}{26} = 57\tfrac{9}{13}$$

$$
\begin{array}{r}
57 \\
26\overline{)1500} \\
130 \\
\hline
200 \\
182 \\
\hline
18 \\
\end{array}
\qquad \frac{18}{26} = \frac{9}{13}
$$

Score = $57\tfrac{9}{13}\%$ (usually rounded to 58%).

238. Outline the steps for expressing a ratio as a percent.

. . . .

Check with page 123, Item 3.

Percent Increase or Decrease

Apply the method of changing ratios to percents to problems dealing with percentage of increase or decrease.

---

239. A patient paid $240 for a private room on the first day at the hospital and $184 on the second day for a semiprivate room. What was the percentage of decrease in the amount of his bill? (Find the amount of the decrease; then divide by the *original* cost.)

. . . .

about 23%

$240 - 184 = 56$ *(amount of decrease)*

$$\frac{56}{240} = x\%$$

$$\frac{7}{30} = \frac{x}{100}$$

$$30x = 700$$

$$x = 23\frac{1}{3}$$

---

240. The number of women in the United States who work rose from about 22 million in 1960 to about 30 million in 1970. What was the percentage of increase? Hint: Find the amount of the increase, then divide by the *original* number.

. . . .

about 36%

Find the increase, then divide by the original number.

$$\frac{8}{22} = x\%$$

$$\frac{4}{11} = \frac{x}{100}$$

$$11x = 400$$

$$x = 36\frac{4}{11}$$

---

241. The number of women holding professional jobs in the United States rose from about 3000 thousand in 1950 to about 4200 thousand in 1970. What was the percentage of increase?

. . . .

40%

$$\frac{1200}{3000} = x\%$$

$$\frac{1200}{3000} = \frac{x}{100}$$

$$\frac{2}{5} = \frac{x}{100}$$

$$x = 40$$

241a.

The number of working wives in the United States increased from 8 million in 1950 to 18 million in 1970. What was the percentage of increase?

. . . .

125%

$$\frac{\overset{5}{\cancel{10}}}{\underset{4}{\cancel{8}}} = \frac{x}{100}$$

$$x = 125$$

---

242. The cost of an antihistamine tablet increased from 3 cents per tablet to 4 cents per tablet. What was the percentage of increase? Find the error in the following incorrect solution and give the correct solution:

$$\frac{1}{4} = x\%$$

$$\frac{1}{4} = \frac{x}{100}$$

$$x = 25$$

. . . .

The percentage of increase is $\dfrac{\text{the increase}}{\text{original price}}$ expressed as a percent. The correct solution is:

$$\frac{1}{3} = x\%$$

$$\frac{1}{3} = \frac{x}{100}$$

$$3x = 100$$

$$x = 33\frac{1}{3}$$

The percentage of increase was actually $33\frac{1}{3}\%$.

243. What are the steps in finding percentage of increase or decrease?

. . . .

Check with page 123, Item 4.

Additional Percent Problems

244. Ten is what percent of 12? (Ten is what part of 12, expressed as a percent?)

. . . .

$83\frac{1}{3}\%$

$$\frac{10}{12} = x\%$$

$$\frac{10}{12} = \frac{x}{100}$$

$$\frac{5}{6} = \frac{x}{100}$$

$$6x = 500$$

$$x = 83\frac{1}{3}$$

10 is $83\frac{1}{3}\%$ of 12

244a.

Eight is what percent of 11?

. . . .

$72\frac{8}{11}\%$

$$\frac{8}{11} = x\%$$

$$\frac{8}{11} = \frac{x}{100}$$

$$11x = 800$$

$$x = 72\frac{8}{11}$$

8 is $72\frac{8}{11}\%$ of 11

245. Twelve is what percent of 10? Notice that the *larger* number is to be considered as a percent of the *smaller* number!

. . . .

120%

$$\frac{12}{10} = \frac{x}{100}$$

$$10x = 1200$$

$$x = 120$$

12 is 120% of 10

245a.

Eleven is what percent of 8?

. . . .

137½%

$$\frac{11}{8} = \frac{x}{100}$$

$$8x = 1100$$

$$x = 137\tfrac{1}{2}$$

11 is 137½% of 8

---

246. Ten is 12% of what? Here the percent is known; the number to which 10 is being compared is the *unknown*.

. . . .

83⅓

$$\frac{10}{x} = 12\%$$

$$\frac{10}{x} = \frac{12}{100}$$

$$12x = 1000$$

$$x = 83\tfrac{1}{3}$$

10 is 12% of 83⅓

246a.

Eight is 11% of what?

. . . .

$72^8/_{11}$

8 is 11% of x

$$\frac{8}{x} = 11\%$$

$$\frac{8}{x} = \frac{11}{100}$$

$$11x = 800$$

$$x = 72^8/_{11}$$

8 is 11% of $72^8/_{11}$

---

247. How many pints (to the nearest pint) is 16% of 5 quarts?

. . . .

2 pints

16% of 5 quarts = 16% of 10 pints =
$$\frac{16}{100} \times 10 = \frac{16}{10} = 1^6/_{10} = 1^3/_5 \text{ pints} =$$
2 pints (to the nearest pint)

247a.

How many inches (to the nearest inch) is 14% of 3 feet?

. . . .

5 inches

14% of 3 feet = 14% of 36 inches =
$$\frac{14}{100} \times 36 = \frac{126}{25} = 5^1/_{25}$$

---

248. Find 2% of 28%.

. . . .

$\dfrac{7}{1250}$

$$\frac{\overset{1}{\cancel{2}}}{\underset{25}{\cancel{100}}} \times \frac{\overset{7}{\cancel{28}}}{\underset{50}{\cancel{100}}} = \frac{7}{1250}$$

248a.

Find 10% of 12%.

. . . .

$\dfrac{3}{250}$

$$\frac{10}{100} \times \frac{12}{100} = \frac{1}{10} \times \frac{3}{25} = \frac{3}{250}$$

249. A bottle contained 5 ounces. This was 22% of the original quantity. How many ounces (to the nearest ounce) were in the original quantity?

. . . .

23 ounces

$$5 = 22\% \text{ of } x; \frac{5}{x} = 22\%$$

$$\frac{5}{x} = \frac{22}{100}$$

$$\frac{5}{x} = \frac{11}{50}$$

$$11x = 250$$

$$x = 22\tfrac{8}{11}$$

249a.

One serving of Popular Cereal provides 1 milligram of iron. This is about 7% of the minimum daily requirement for iron. What is the minimum daily requirement for iron?

. . . .

About 14 milligrams

$$1 = 7\% \text{ of } x$$

$$\frac{1}{x} = 7\%$$

$$\frac{1}{x} = \frac{7}{100}$$

$$7x = 1 \times 100$$

$$7x = 100$$

$$x = 14\tfrac{2}{7}$$

SUMMARY

1. The symbol % tells you: "divide by 100"; alternatives are "per hundred" or "in a hundred."

   Examples: $25\% = \dfrac{25}{100}, \dfrac{1}{2}\% = \dfrac{\frac{1}{2}}{100} = \dfrac{1}{200}$

2. To find $x\%$ of any number, multiply the number by x and divide by 100.

   Example: 5% of $72 = \dfrac{5}{100} \times 72 = \dfrac{18}{5} = 3\dfrac{3}{5}$

3. To change any number, N, to a percent, set up the proportion $N = {}^{x}/_{100}$; solve for x, then $N = x\%$.

   Example: Suppose $N = \dfrac{3}{5} = x\%$

   $\dfrac{3}{5} = \dfrac{x}{100}, x = 60$

   $\dfrac{3}{5} = 60\%$

4. To find the percentage of increase (or decrease) find the amount of increase (or decrease), divide by the *original* number and change to percent.

   Example: Suppose a price is raised from 50 cents to 60 cents.

   $\dfrac{\text{amount of increase}}{\text{original number}} = \dfrac{10}{50} = \dfrac{1}{5} = 20\%$

   Suppose a price is decreased from 60 cents to 50 cents.

   $\dfrac{\text{amount of decrease}}{\text{original number}} = \dfrac{10}{60} = \dfrac{1}{6} = 16\dfrac{2}{3}\%$

EXERCISES FOR EXTRA PRACTICE

1. Change to mixed numbers, whole numbers, or common fractions. Simplify.

   (a) 18%   (b) 5%   (c) 400%   (d) 1000%   (e) $\frac{1}{10}$%

   (f) $\frac{1}{4}$%   (g) $3\frac{1}{2}$%   (h) 350%

2. Find the following quantities. In each case consider whether your result is reasonable.

   (a) 5% of 8 ounces   (b) 20% of 10 ounces   (c) 25% of 2 grams

   (d) 15% of 4 liters   (e) 40% of 10 pounds   (f) 200% of $3

   (g) $\frac{1}{2}$% of 10 inches

3. Change to percentages.

   (a) 5   (b) 48   (c) 100   (d) 1   (e) $\frac{1}{2}$

   (f) $3\frac{1}{2}$ (g) $\frac{3}{4}$ (h) $\frac{5}{8}$ (i) $\frac{2}{5}$ (j) $\frac{3}{20}$

4. Assume a raise in wages from $250 to $300. Find the percentage of increase.

5. Assume a decrease in quantity from 32 ounces to 28 ounces. Find the percentage of decrease.

. . . .

Answers

1. (a) $\frac{9}{50}$ (b) $\frac{1}{20}$ (c) 4   (d) 10   (e) $\frac{1}{1000}$

   (f) $\frac{1}{400}$ (g) $\frac{7}{200}$ (h) $3\frac{1}{2}$

2. (a) $\frac{2}{5}$ ounce   (b) 2 ounces   (c) $\frac{1}{2}$ gram   (d) $\frac{3}{5}$ liter

   (e) 4 pounds   (f) $6   (g) $\frac{1}{20}$ inch

3. (a) 500%   (b) 4800%   (c) 10,000%   (d) 100%
   (e) 50%   (f) 350%   (g) 75%

   (h) $62\frac{1}{2}$%   (i) 40%   (j) 15%

4. 20%   5. $12\frac{1}{2}$%

INVENTORY

The set of exercises below will show you whether you are already an expert or whether you need a little more practice. If you do need more practice, the numbers next to the answers below will direct you to the particular frames that should receive your special attention.

1. Change to mixed numbers or common fractions and simplify as much as possible: 52%, 7$\frac{9}{10}$%, $\frac{4}{1000}$%, 325%, $\frac{3}{4}$%.

2. A flask contains 22 ounces of a 5% sodium bicarbonate solution. How many ounces of sodium bicarbonate are in the flask?

3. Mrs. Moneybags reported that $7420 worth of jewelry had been stolen. The police recovered 80% of the missing jewelry. What percentage of the jewelry was still missing and what was its value?

4. Change to percents: $\frac{213}{1000}$, $\frac{1}{16}$, 2$\frac{1}{2}$, 1$\frac{17}{20}$, 350.

5. Just in time for Mother's Day: cool, easy-care dacron and cotton negligees, on sale for $21, regularly $28. What is the percent reduction?

6. What percent of 10 is 12?

. . . .

Answers

1. 51% = $\frac{13}{25}$, 7$\frac{9}{10}$% = $\frac{79}{1000}$, $\frac{4}{1000}$% = $\frac{1}{25,000}$, 325% = $\frac{13}{4}$ or 3$\frac{1}{4}$, $\frac{3}{4}$% = $\frac{3}{400}$
   (Frames 204—217)

2. 1$\frac{1}{10}$ (Frames 218—228)

3. 20%; $1484 (Frames 218—228)

4. 21$\frac{3}{10}$%, 6$\frac{1}{4}$%, 250%, 185%, 35,000% (Frames 229—238)

5. 25% (Frames 239—243)

6. 120% (Frames 244—249)

If your answers are correct, proceed to Section 6. Otherwise, study the relevant frames, and then go back to the Proficiency Gauge on page 101.

DECIMAL FRACTIONS AND MIXED DECIMALS

The thermometer records a patient's temperature as 103.1°F. A doctor's order calls for atropine sulfate 0.4 mg. The label on the stock bottle of digoxin reads 1 cc. = 0.5 mg. During a blood transfusion, a patient improves after receiving 2.9 pints of blood. Another patient is poisoned by a dose of 5 grams of a drug instead of 0.05 grams. (Death may result from misplacement of a decimal point!) There is hardly a day in the life of a nurse when she does not need decimal fractions in or out of the hospital. Measurements are more often expressed as decimal fractions rather than common fractions because they simplify the process of computation.

Upon completion of this section, the student should be able to:

1. Read and write numbers in decimal form.

2. Change a decimal fraction to a common fraction or the reverse.

3. Arrange a set of mixed decimals in order of magnitude.

4. Add, subtract, multiply, and divide mixed decimals.

5. Round an answer.

6. Express a given percent as a mixed decimal.

7. Change any mixed decimal to a percent.

PROFICIENCY GAUGE

To gauge your proficiency in using decimal numbers, work out the following exercises. Uncover the printed answers only after you have answered all the questions.

1. Write in words: 31.67 inches.

2. Write as a mixed number: 20.03.

3. Write as a decimal fraction: (a) 4 hundredths degrees (b) $\frac{5}{1000}$ mile

4. Arrange in order of size, the smallest first: 0.01, 0.0001, 0.10, 1.001, 1.101.

5. Add: 2.1 + 3.002 + 0.21.

6. Subtract: 21.35 − 2.001.

7. Multiply: 0.037 by 100; divide 4.35 by 10.

8. Multiply: 3.013 by 91.

9. Divide 0.0174 by 6.

10. Divide 12 by 5 and express the answer as a mixed decimal.

11. Divide 1.6 by 0.32.

12. Express $\frac{2}{11}$ as a 2-place decimal fraction.

13. Change the following to decimals: 52%, 7.9%, 0.004%.

14. Change to percents: 0.213, 2.01, 354.2.

. . . .

Answers

1. Thirty-one and sixty-seven hundredths inches

2. $20^3/_{100}$

3. (a) 0.04 degree; (b) 0.005 mile

4. 0.0001, 0.01, 0.10, 1.001, 1.101

5. 5.312

6. 19.349

7. 3.7; 0.435

8. 274.183

9. 0.0029

10. 2.4

11. 5

12. 0.18

13. 0.52, 0.079, 0.00004

14. 21.3%, 201%, 35,420%

If you have errors, go on to Frame 250. Otherwise skip ahead to Section 7.

Read page 3 for instructions if you have not already done so.

Meaning of Decimal Fractions

250. What would you say is distinctive about the following set of fractions:

$$\frac{76}{10}, \frac{3}{10}, \frac{7}{10}, \frac{89}{100}, \frac{17}{1000}, \frac{63}{100}, \frac{731}{10,000}, \frac{1}{10}.$$

. . . .

The denominators are all related to 10. We call these special denominators (10, 10 × 10, 10 × 10 × 10, etc.) powers of 10.

---

251. Write five common fractions whose denominators are different powers of 10.

. . . .

There are many different possibilities. One might write the following set:

$$\frac{1}{10}, \frac{3}{100}, \frac{8}{1000}, \frac{79}{10,000}, \frac{852}{100,000}.$$

---

252. Use a proportion to change ¾ to a fraction with a denominator of 100.

. . . .

$$\frac{75}{100}$$

$$\frac{3}{4} = \frac{x}{100}$$

$$4x = 300$$

$$x = 75$$

$$\frac{3}{4} = \frac{75}{100}$$

---

253. Change ⅛ to a fraction with a denominator of 1000.

. . . .

$$\frac{125}{1000}$$

$$\frac{1}{8} = \frac{x}{1000}$$

$$8x = 1000$$

$$x = 125$$

$$\frac{1}{8} = \frac{125}{1000}$$

254. All fractions can be expressed exactly or approximately as fractions with denominators which are powers of 10. For instance, $\frac{9}{80} = \frac{1125}{10,000}$ and $\frac{1}{3}$ is approximately equal to $\frac{33}{100}$. Since 100 and 10,000 are numbers that are easy to compute with, a whole system of measurement has been built up around them. Write all the proper fractions with a denominator of 10.

. . . .

$$\frac{1}{10}, \frac{2}{10}, \frac{3}{10}, \frac{4}{10}, \frac{5}{10}, \frac{6}{10}, \frac{7}{10}, \frac{8}{10}, \frac{9}{10}$$

255. Each proper fraction with a denominator of 10 may be written more simply as 0.1, 0.2, 0.3, _____ , 0.5, _____, 0.7 _____, _____. What has replaced the denominator? What symbol emphasizes that we are dealing with a proper fraction?

. . . .

0.4, 0.6, 0.8, 0.9; the *decimal point* has replaced the denominator 10. The 0 in front of the decimal point shows that we are talking about proper fractions only.

256. A decimal fraction is equivalent to a common fraction whose denominator is _____.

. . . .

Check with page 162, Item 1.

Decimal Places

257. Complete the following table:

Common Fraction	Equivalent Decimal Fraction	In Words
$\frac{1}{100}$	0.01	one hundredth
$\frac{7}{100}$	0.07	seven hundredths
$\frac{9}{100}$		
$\frac{23}{100}$	0.23	twenty-three hundredths
$\frac{37}{100}$		
$\frac{50}{100}$		
	0.03	
	0.49	
	0.90	

. . . .

$\frac{9}{100} = 0.09$ nine hundredths

$\frac{37}{100} = 0.37$ thirty-seven hundredths

$\frac{50}{100} = 0.50$ fifty hundredths

$\frac{3}{100} = 0.03$ three hundredths

$\frac{49}{100} = 0.49$ forty-nine hundredths

$\frac{90}{100} = 0.90$ ninety hundredths

258. Three-place decimals—complete the table:

Common Fraction	Equivalent Decimal Fraction	In Words
$\dfrac{1}{1000}$	0.001	one thousandth
$\dfrac{2}{1000}$		
$\dfrac{23}{1000}$		
$\dfrac{427}{1000}$	0.427	four hundred twenty-seven thousandths
$\dfrac{391}{1000}$		

. . . .

$\dfrac{2}{1000} = 0.002$ two thousandths

$\dfrac{23}{1000} = 0.023$ twenty-three thousandths

$\dfrac{391}{1000} = 0.391$ three hundred ninety-one thousandths

259. On Monday, June 10, the *New York Times* reported the following standings of base-ball teams: Los Angeles 0.582, Pittsburgh 0.500, Boston 0.510. What are the common fraction equivalents of these scores?

. . . .

$\dfrac{582}{1000}, \dfrac{500}{1000}, \dfrac{510}{1000}$

259a.

Write the common fraction equivalent of the following decimal fractions: 0.007, 0.053, 0.973.

. . . .

$\dfrac{7}{1000}, \dfrac{53}{1000}, \dfrac{973}{1000}$

260. Wherever numbers appear in words in the following statement, change to common fractions and to decimal fractions:

To write the Kinsey report, interviewers gathered information from a large group of people. Of this group, six-tenths were college graduates, twenty-six hundredths were graduate students, sixteen-thousandths were from the underworld, five-thousandths were business executives, eight-tenths were Protestants.

. . . .

To write the Kinsey report, interviewers gathered information from a large group of people. Of this group, $\frac{6}{10}$ (0.6) were college graduates, $\frac{26}{100}$ (0.26) were graduate students, $\frac{16}{1000}$ (0.016) were from the underworld, $\frac{5}{1000}$ (0.005) were business executives, $\frac{8}{10}$ (0.8) were Protestants.

261. Complete the following table:

Common Fraction	Number of Zeros in Denominator	Number of Decimal Places	Decimal Fraction
$\frac{37}{100}$	2	2	0.37
$\frac{7}{1000}$	3	3	0.007
$\frac{9}{10}$			
$\frac{9}{100}$			
			0.00007

. . . .

$\frac{9}{10}$	1	1	0.9
$\frac{9}{100}$	2	2	0.09
$\frac{7}{100,000}$	5	5	0.00007

262. The number of zeros in the denominator of $^2/_{100,000}$ is _____. Write as decimal fraction: $^2/_{100,000}$.

. . . .

5 zeros; 0.00002 (5 places to the right of the decimal point)

262a.

Write $^{33}/_{100,000,000}$ as a decimal fraction.

. . . .

0.00000033 (8 decimal places corresponding to the 8 zeros in the denominator of the fraction)

262b.

How many zeros are there in the denominator of the common fraction corresponding to the decimal fraction 0.37215? Write the equivalent common fraction.

. . . .

5; $\dfrac{37215}{100,000}$

---

263. The number of decimal places in a decimal fraction corresponds to the number of _____ in the denominator of the equivalent common fraction.

. . . .

Check page 162, Item 2.

264. Complete the following table:

Decimal Fractions	Common Fractions
0.10034	$\dfrac{10034}{100,000}$
0.354162	
0.076	
0.2105	
	$\dfrac{607}{10,000}$
	$\dfrac{3}{1000}$

· · · · · · · · · · · ·

$0.354162 = \dfrac{354,162}{1,000,000}$

$0.076 \quad = \dfrac{76}{1000}$

$0.2105 \quad = \dfrac{2,105}{10,000}$

$0.0607 \quad = \dfrac{607}{10,000}$

$0.003 \quad = \dfrac{3}{1000}$

Inserting Zeros in a Decimal Fraction

265. Change 0.3 to a 4-place decimal.

· · · · · · · · · · · ·

0.3000   *Since* $\dfrac{3}{10} = \dfrac{3000}{10,000}$, *then 0.3 = 0.3000.*

265a.

Change 0.012 to a 5-place decimal.

· · · · · · · · · · · ·

0.01200   Since $\frac{12}{1000} = \frac{1200}{100,000}$, $0.012 = 0.01200$.

265b.

Change 0.93 to a 6-place decimal.

. . . .

0.930000

---

266. Change 0.012 to a 4-place decimal.

. . . .

0.0120

---

267. Change 0.2300 to a 2-place decimal.

. . . .

0.23

267a.

Change 0.30100 to a 3-place decimal.

. . . .

0.301

267b.

Change 0.001200 to a 4-place decimal.

. . . .

0.0012

---

268. Change 0.003400 to a 4-place decimal.

. . . .

0.0034

268a.

Change 0.010 to a 4-place decimal.

. . . .

0.0100

269. Change 0.0870 to a 6-place decimal.

. . . .

0.087000

270. Write as common fractions and simplify: 0.7, 0.70, 0.700, 0.7000. Which is the greatest, if any?

. . . .

$0.7 = \dfrac{7}{10}$, $0.70 = \dfrac{70}{100} = \dfrac{7}{10}$, $0.700 = \dfrac{700}{1000} = \dfrac{7}{10}$, etc.

all equal

271. The value of the decimal fraction is unchanged if we place zeros (directly to the right of the decimal point/directly to the right of the last digit); e.g., 0.325 (is equal to/is unequal to) 0.325000 and 0.325 (is equal to/is unequal to) 0.00325.

. . . .

The value of the decimal fraction is *unchanged* if we place zeros *directly to the right of the last digit*. For example, 0.325 is equal to 0.32500, but 0.325 is *not* equal to 0.00325.

271a.

Using zeros, write a decimal fraction with 7 decimal places equivalent to 0.98.

. . . .

0.9800000

Two decimal places are given. To make a 7-place number without changing the value, simply place 5 zeros to the right of 0.98.

272. What happens to the value of a decimal fraction if 0 is inserted directly to the right of the decimal point? What happens to the value of a decimal fraction if 0 is inserted directly to the right of the last digit?

. . . .

Check page 162, Item 3.

Relative Size

The following frames explain how to tell relative sizes of decimal fractions by converting to the same number of decimal places.

273. (a) 0.9 (is equal to/greater than/less than) 0.9000.
     (b) 0.9 (is equal to/greater than/less than) 0.0009.

. . . .

(a) 0.9 is equal to 0.9000.

(a) $0.9 = \frac{9}{10}$, and $0.9000 = \frac{9000}{10,000} = \frac{9}{10}$

(b) 0.9 is greater than 0.0009.

(b) $0.9 = \frac{9}{10} = \frac{9000}{10,000}$ and $0.0009 = \frac{9}{10,000}$

Since $\frac{9000}{10,000}$ is greater than $\frac{9}{10,000}$, 0.9 is greater than 0.0009.

274. Which is greater, 0.3 or 0.007? Hint: Change 0.3 to a 3-place decimal.

. . . .

0.3 = 0.300. 0.300 is greater than 0.007 because $\frac{300}{1000}$ is greater than $\frac{7}{1000}$.

274a.

Which is greater, 0.5 or 0.05?

. . . .

0.5 is greater than 0.05.

To compare 0.5 with 0.05, change 0.5 to 0.50 so that both numbers have the same number of decimal places; then, 0.50 is greater than 0.05 because $^{50}/_{100}$ is greater than $^{5}/_{100}$.

274b.

Which is greater, 0.012 or 0.12?

. . . .

0.12 is greater than 0.012.

Change 0.12 to 0.120 so that both numbers have the same number of decimal places; then 0.120 (or $^{120}/_{1000}$) is greater than 0.012 (or $^{12}/_{1000}$).

Addition or Subtraction

275. Nurse Ann Kompatent needed three different solutions into which she poured the following quantities of atropine: 0.052 milligrams, 0.8 milligrams, and 0.12 milligrams. What was the total amount of atropine used?

. . . .

$$\begin{array}{r} 0.052 \\ 0.800 \\ +0.120 \\ \hline 0.972 \end{array}$$

Using common fractions, the computation would be:

$$\frac{52}{1000} + \frac{8}{10} + \frac{12}{100} = \frac{52}{1000} + \frac{800}{1000} + \frac{120}{1000}$$

276. When adding or subtracting common fractions with unlike denominators, we first write out equivalent fractions with like denominators. When adding or subtracting decimal fractions with an unequal number of decimal places, we equalize the number of decimal places by _____.

. . . .

adding zeros

277. Add: 0.2, 0.05, 0.111. Subtract: 0.05 from 0.2.

. . . .

$$\begin{array}{r} 0.200 \\ 0.050 \\ +0.111 \\ \hline 0.361 \end{array} \qquad \begin{array}{r} 0.20 \\ - \ 0.05 \\ \hline 0.15 \end{array}$$

278. Mr. Strong's heart is in a weakened condition. He has been given two doses of a $\frac{1}{1000}$ solution of epinephrine as a stimulant, but the amount of drug administered must be watched carefully to prevent death from this powerful drug. The first dose given was 0.03 milliliters and the second dose was 0.045 milliliters. How many milliliters has he received so far?

. . . .

0.075 milliliters

278a.

Mrs. Mater, Mrs. Maman, and Mrs. Mère, patients on the obstetric ward, were given subcutaneous injections of scopolamine hydrobromide in dosages of 0.3 milligrams, 0.4 milligrams, and 0.06 milligrams. Find the total amount of drug used.

. . . .

0.76 milligrams.

278b.

Add 0.29 and 0.73 and check by changing to common fractions.

. . . .

$$
\begin{array}{r}
0.29 \\
+\,0.73 \\
\hline
1.02
\end{array}
\qquad\qquad
\frac{29}{100} + \frac{73}{100} = \frac{102}{100} = 1\frac{2}{100}
$$

---

279. Subtract 0.31 from 0.542 and check by addition.

. . . .

$$
\begin{array}{r}
0.542 \\
-\,0.310 \\
\hline
0.232
\end{array}
\qquad\qquad
\begin{array}{r}
0.232 \\
+\,0.310 \\
\hline
0.542
\end{array}
$$

---

280. Outline the procedure for adding and subtracting decimal fractions.

. . . .

Check page 162, Item 4.

281. Mixed numbers in decimal form, e.g., 1.02 in Frame 278b above, are called mixed decimals. Complete the table:

Mixed Number	Mixed Decimal	In Words
$1\frac{9}{10}$	1.9	one *and* 9 tenths (one-point-nine)
$23\frac{7}{100}$	23.07	twenty-three *and* seven hundredths (or two-three point-oh-seven)
$49\frac{29}{1000}$		
	3.102	

What spoken word indicates the position of the decimal?

. . . .

It is important to remember that the position of the decimal is indicated, when speaking, by "and."

$49\frac{29}{1000} = 49.029$ forty-nine and twenty-nine thousandths (or four-nine-point-oh-two-nine)

$3\frac{102}{1000} = 3.102$ three and one hundred two thousandths (or three-point-one-oh-two)

282. Write in decimal form: (a) five hundred thirty-seven thousandths; (b) five hundred and thirty-seven thousandths.

. . . .

(a) 0.537; (b) 500.037

283. Write in words: 200.002; 0.202; 0.0202; and 202.02.

. . . .

two hundred and two thousandths; two hundred two thousandths; two hundred two ten-thousandths; two hundred two and two hundredths.

284. Add the numbers given in Frame 283.

. . . .

200.0020
0.2020
0.0202
202.0200
402.2442

285. Sustained muscular relaxation was produced in Mr. Atlas by continuous drip infu-
sion of anectine chloride in which approximately 2.5 milligrams were given the first
minute, 2.45 milligrams were given the second minute, 2.45 milligrams were given
the third minute, 2.5 milligrams were given the fourth minute, and 2.47 milligrams
were given the fifth minute. Approximately how many milligrams were given all
together?

. . . .

12.37

286. An infant measured 19.75 inches at birth. One month later, he was 21.25 inches.
How much had he grown? (Check your result.)

. . . .

21.25   *Check:* *19.75*
−19.75   *1.50*
   1.50 inches   *21.25*

287. Initially, a patient received an oral dose of 1.5 milligrams of his special medicine.
In the next three days, he received 0.5 milligrams, 0.4 milligrams, and 0.25 milligrams. How much is left from the original supply of 3.5 milligrams?

. . . .

0.85 milligrams   *Used*
                          1.50
                          0.50
                          0.40   *3.50*
                          0.25   *−2.65*
                          2.65   *0.85*

Multiplication by Powers of Ten

288. Multiply each of the following decimal fractions by 10 and compare the result with the original fraction:

Original Decimal Fraction	Common Fraction Equivalent × 10	Result in Decimal Form
0.70		7 or 7.0
0.007	$\frac{7}{1000} \times 10^1 = \frac{7}{100}$	0.07
0.07		

In each case the result of multiplying by 10 can be obtained simply by moving the decimal point _____ place to the right.

. . . .

0.70	$\frac{7}{10} \times 10 = 7$	7 or 7.0
0.07	$\frac{7}{100} \times 10 = \frac{7}{10}$	0.7

To multiply by 10 move the decimal point *one* place to the right.

---

289. Use the shortcut to multiply by 10:

0.91 × 10 = _____

1.805 × 10 = _____

23.001 × 10 = _____

. . . .

0.91 × 10 = 9.1

1.805 × 10 = 18.05

23.001 × 10 = 230.01

289a.

10.012   × 10 = _____

0.00034 × 10 = _____

. . . .

10.012   × 10 = 100.12
0.00034 × 10 =   0.0034

---

290. For each of the following quantities of sodium contained in different solutions, find the total quantity in 10 such solutions:
(a) 0.02512   (b) 25.12   (c) 2512   (d) 0.2512   (e) 251.2   (f) 2.512

. . . .

Multiply each number by 10:
(a) 0.2512   (b) 251.2   (c) 25,120   (d) 2.512   (e) 2512.0   (f) 25.12

---

291. Each time we multiply by 10, we move the decimal point one place to the right. Multiplying by 100 is the same as multiplying by 10 and then by 10 a second time. To multiply by 100 requires moving the decimal point_____ places to the right.

71.235 × 100 = _____

. . . .

two; 7123.5

---

292. Multiplying by 1000 is equivalent to multiplying by 10, once, then by 10 again, then by 10 a third time. Therefore, to multiply by 1000 move the decimal point _____ places to the right.

. . . .

three

---

293. 3.1416 ×   1,000 = _____
20.03   ×   100 = _____
0.03   ×   10,000 = _____
0.0374 × 100,000 = _____

. . . .

3141.6
2003.0
 300.0
3740.0

Division by Powers of Ten

294. Divide each of the following decimal fractions by 10 and compare the result with the original fraction:

Original Decimal Fraction	Common Fraction Equivalent ÷ 10	Result in Decimal Form
0.72	$\frac{72}{100} \div 10 =$ $\frac{72}{100} \times \frac{1}{10} = \frac{72}{1000}$	0.072
0.9	$\frac{9}{10} \div 10 = \frac{9}{10} \times \frac{1}{10} = \frac{9}{100}$	0.09
0.21		

In each case the result of dividing by 10 can be obtained simply by moving the decimal _____ place to the _____ .

. . . .

$$0.21 = \frac{21}{100} \div 10 = \frac{21}{100} \times \frac{1}{10} = \frac{21}{1000} = 0.021$$

To divide by 10, move the decimal point *one* place to the *left*.

295. Use the shortcut to divide by 10:

$0.91 \div 10 =$ _____

$1.805 \div 10 =$ _____

$23.001 \div 10 =$ _____

. . . .

$0.91 \div 10 = 0.091$

$1.805 \div 10 = 0.1805$

$23.001 \div 10 = 2.3001$

Move the decimal point one place to the left.

295a.

$10.012 \div 10 =$ _____

$0.00034 \div 10 =$ _____

. . . .

10.012   ÷ 10 = 1.0012

0.00034 ÷ 10 = 0.000034

---

296. Suppose you have 71.3 grams of powder and must make up 10 doses from this supply. How many grams would you put in each dose?

. . . .

71.3 ÷ 10 = 7.13 grams

---

297. Each time we divide by 10, we move the decimal point one place to the left. Dividing by 100 is the same as dividing by 10 and then by 10 a second time. To divide by 100, move the decimal point _____ place(s) to the _____. For example, 712.35 ÷ 100 = _____ .

. . . .

To divide by 100, move the decimal point *two* places to the *left*.
712.35 ÷ 100 = 7.1235.

---

298. Divide 63.72 by 10, by 100, by 1000.

. . . .

6.372, 0.6372, 0.06372

---

299. There are 49.32 grams of sodium in 100 cc. of solution. How many grams of sodium are there per cc.?

. . . .

0.4932

---

300. Division by 10, 100, or 1000 is accomplished by moving the decimal point _____, _____, or _____ places to the LEFT. The resulting number is (less than/greater than) the original number.

. . . .

Division by 10, 100, 1000, etc., is accomplished by moving the decimal point 1, 2, 3, etc., places to the LEFT. The quotient is a number that is LESS than the original number.

301. Complete the following table:

Operation	State How to Move Decimal Point	Compare Result with Original Number
multiply by 10	one place to *right*	*greater*
divide by 10	one place to *left*	*less*
divide by 100		
multiply by 100		
multiply by 1000		
divide by 1000		

. . . .

divide by 100	two places to left	less
multiply by 100	two places to right	greater
multiply by 1000	three places to right	greater
divide by 1000	three places to left	less

302. In division by powers of 10, the decimal point is moved to the _____;
the result is L _ _ _ than the original number.

	Multiply by 100	Divide by 1000
321.257		
751.2		
1.257		

. . . .

In division by powers of 10, the decimal point is moved to the LEFT; the result
is LESS than the original number.

321.257	32,125.7	0.321257
751.2	75,120.0	0.7512
1.257	125.7	0.001257

303. Express 2.5% as a decimal.

. . . .

0.025   *2.5% = 2.5 ÷ 100 = 0.025*

303a.

Express 34.25% as a decimal.

. . . .

0.3425   *34.25% = 34.25 ÷ 100 = 0.3425*

---

304. Express 0.001% as a decimal.

. . . .

0.00001   *0.001 ÷ 100 = 0.00001*

304a.

Express 1.01% as a decimal.

. . . .

0.0101   *1.01% = 1.01 ÷ 100 = 0.0101*

---

305. Express the ratio 0.2 : 10 as a decimal, then as a ratio with no decimals.

. . . .

0.02, 2 : 100   *0.2 : 10 = 0.2 ÷ 10 = 0.02*

305a.

Express the ratio 0.05 : 1000 as a decimal, then as a ratio with no decimals.

. . . .

0.00005, 5 : 100,000   *0.05 : 1000 = 0.05 ÷ 1000 = 0.00005 =*

$$\frac{5}{100,000} \text{ or } \frac{1}{20,000}$$

306. Find x if $2.5 = x\%$.

. . . .

$x = 250$

$$2.5 = \frac{x}{100}$$

Multiply both sides by 100.

$x = 2.5 \times 100$

$x = 250$

$2.5 = 250\%$

306a.

Find x if $11.9 = x\%$.

. . . .

$x = 1190$

$$11.9 = \frac{x}{100}$$

$x = 11.9 \times 100$

$x = 1190$

$11.9 = 1190\%$

---

307. Find x in each case:

(a) $0.21 = x\%$ (Express 0.21 as a percent.)

(b) $0.21\% = x$ (Express 0.21% as a decimal fraction.)

. . . .

(a) $x = 21$

(b) $x = 0.0021$

(a) $0.21 = \frac{x}{100}$; $x = 21$

(b) $x = \frac{0.21}{100}$; $x = 0.0021$

307a.

Find x:

(a) $0.03 = x\%$

(b) $0.03\% = x$

. . . .

(a) $0.03 = \dfrac{x}{100}$, $x = 3$

(b) $0.03\% = \dfrac{0.03}{100} = 0.0003$

---

308. Find x:

   (a) $0.327 = x\%$

   (b) $0.327\% = x$

. . . .

   (a) $\dfrac{0.327}{1} = \dfrac{x}{100}$

   $x = 32.7$

   $0.327 = 32.7\%$

   (b) $\dfrac{0.327}{100} = x$

   $x = 0.00327$

308a.

Find x:

   (a) $0.732 = x\%$

   (b) $0.732\% = x$

. . . .

   (a) $\dfrac{0.732}{1} = \dfrac{x}{100}$

   $x = 73.2$

   (b) $\dfrac{0.732}{100} = x = .00732$

Multiplication of Mixed Decimals

---

309. Each cc. of alcohol weighs 0.79 gram. What is the weight of 3 cc. of alcohol?

. . . .

2.37 grams   *3 cc. contains 0.79 + 0.79 + 0.79 grams*
                                = 2.37 grams, or 3 × 0.79 = 2.37 grams

---

310. Chlormerodrin is available in 18.3 milligram tablets for use in many types of edema. The doctor prescribes 4 tablets daily. How many milligrams of chlormerodrin is the patient receiving daily?

. . . .

73.2 milligrams   *4 X 18.3 = 73.2*

---

311. If $\dfrac{2}{10} \times \dfrac{3}{10} = \dfrac{6}{100}$, then 0.2 X 0.3 = _____ .

. . . .

0.06

311a.

If $\dfrac{2}{100} \times \dfrac{3}{1000} = \dfrac{6}{100,000}$, then 0.02 X 0.003 = _____ .

. . . .

0.00006

---

312. Refer to Frame 311. Multiplying 0.2 by 0.3 is equivalent to multiplying 2 by 3 (the numerators) and then dividing by 100. To divide decimals by 100, we move the decimal point _____ places to the left.

. . . .

two   *2 X 3 = 6*

and $0.2 \times 0.3 = \dfrac{2}{10} \times \dfrac{3}{10} = \dfrac{2 \times 3}{10 \times 10}$

$= \dfrac{6}{100} = 0.06$

The product of a 1-place decimal and a 1-place decimal is a 2-place decimal.

---

313. Multiplying 0.02 by 0.003 is equivalent to multiplying 2 by 3 and then moving the decimal point _____ places to the left.

. . . .

five

$2 \times 3 = 6$

but $0.02 \times 0.003 = 0.00006$

since $0.02 \times 0.003 = \dfrac{2}{100} \times \dfrac{3}{1000} =$

$\dfrac{2 \times 3}{100 \times 1000} = \dfrac{6}{100,000} = 0.00006$

The product of a 2-place decimal and a 3-place decimal is a 5-place decimal.

313a.

Multiplying 21.21 by 2.056 is equivalent to multiplying 2121 by 2056 and then marking off _____ decimal places.

. . . .

five

---

314. Given that $23 \times 451 = 10,373$, find 0.23×4.51.

. . . .

1.0373

---

315. Find 23.1×0.3.

. . . .

6.93

$231 \times 3 = 693$, then mark off two decimal places.

315a.

Find 0.2×0.01.

. . . .

0.002

$2 \times 1 = 2$, then mark off three decimal places.

---

316. Place the decimal point properly in each of the following answers:

   2.53 × 15   = 3795

   42.3 × 0.2 = 846

   0.61 × 0.72 = 04392

   0.31 × 0.03 = 93

   . . . .

   2.53 × 15   = 37.95

   42.3 × 0.2 = 8.46

   0.61 × 0.72 = 0.4392

   0.31 × 0.03 = 0.0093

317. Multiply:

   0.03 × 15 = _____

   0.8 ×   5 = _____

   0.09 × 10 = _____

   1.98 × 100 = _____

   . . . .

0.45	*0.03 × 15 = 0.45*
4	*0.8 × 5 = 4.0*
0.9	*0.09 × 10 = 0.9 (move decimal point 1 place to right)*
198	*1.98 × 100 = 198 (move decimal point 2 places to right)*

318. A bank pays 5.67% per annum. If you keep $21.50 in the bank for 1 year, how much interest should you receive? (Change 5.67% to a decimal and multiply by 21.50.)

   . . . .

   $1.22 $5.67\% = \dfrac{5.67}{100} = 0.0567$

   $$\begin{array}{r} 567 \\ 2150 \\ \hline 28350 \\ 567 \\ 1134 \\ \hline 1.219050 \end{array}$$

319. It has been estimated that the cost of daily patient care in hospitals is likely to rise more than 35% in the next 5 years. If the cost now is $140.95, about how much higher is the cost expected to be 5 years from now, and what will the cost be then?

. . . .

more than $190.28

$140.95 $ 49.33 higher
      .35
    70475 $140.95
    42285 $ 49.33
$49.3325 $190.28

More than $49.33 higher

320. The daily food ration that an astronaut is given is equivalent to about 2600 calories. If the normal albumin content of the rations is supplemented by 17% of the total calorie value, what is the calorie value of the supplement?

. . . .

442 calories

2600
 .17
18200
2600
442.00

321. How many pints (to the nearest pint) is 16% of 5 quarts?

. . . .

2 pints

5 quarts = 10 pints
0.16 × 10 = 1.6 (almost 2)

321a.

The minimum daily requirement for vitamin C is 30 milligrams. Sta-helthy vitamin capsules contain 125% of the minimum daily requirement for vitamin C. How many milligrams of vitamin C are in each capsule?

. . . .

37.5 milligrams

125% × 30 = 1.25 × 30 = 37.5 milligrams

322. Find 2% of 28%. Express your result as a percent.

. . . .

0.56%   *2% of 28% = 2% × 28% = 0.02 × 0.28*
$$= 0.0056 = \frac{0.56}{100}$$

323. Find 0.9 of 1% (necessary in preparation of normal saline solutions).

. . . .

0.009   *0.9 of 1% = 0.9 × 0.01 = 0.009*

324. Outline the procedure for multiplying mixed decimals.

. . . .

Check page 162, Item 6.

Division of Mixed Decimals

325. A total of 2.44 ounces of medicine are to be given in 4 equal doses. How many ounces are there per dose? Check by multiplying the answer by 4.

. . . .

$$\begin{array}{r} 0.61 \\ 4\overline{)2.44} \end{array}$$ *Check: 4 × 0.61 = 2.44*

326. Divide and check: $5\overline{)74.035}$; $71\overline{)22.294}$.

. . . .

$$\begin{array}{r} 14.807 \\ 5\overline{)74.035} \end{array}$$ *Check: 5 × 14.807 = 74.035*

$$\begin{array}{r} 0.314 \\ 71\overline{)22.294} \\ \underline{21.3} \\ 99 \\ \underline{71} \\ 284 \\ \underline{284} \end{array}$$ *Check: 71 × 0.314 = 22.294*

327. To relieve severe edema, the doctor prescribes a daily dose of 96.085 milligrams of chlormerodrin. Available tablets contain 18.3 milligrams. Estimate how many tablets you should administer to the patient every day if you were the nurse.

. . . .

5

To estimate, round 96.085 and 18.3 to 96 and 18. Consider how many sets of 18 milligrams there are in 96 milligrams.

$$\frac{96}{18} = 5\frac{1}{3}$$

---

328. *Estimate* the answer, then place the decimal point properly in each of the following equations: $9.78 \div 3 = 326$; $143.91 \div 12.3 = 117$.

. . . .

3.26

11.7

9 ÷ 3 = 3 (estimate)

144 ÷ 12 = 12 (estimate)

---

329. To find the exact answer to the question in Frame 327, we must divide:

$$18.3\overline{)96.075}$$

To learn how to treat the decimal points, rewrite this division as a ratio:

$$\frac{96.075}{18.3}$$

Multiply numerator and denominator by 10:

$$\frac{960.75}{183}$$

Rewrite as a long division problem in which the divisor is a whole number:

```
        5.25
183 ) 960.75
      915
       45 7
       36 6
        9 15
        9 15
```

How have the decimal points been moved in the numerator and denominator?

. . . .

One place to the right in the denominator (18.3 to 183) and one place to the right in the numerator (96.085 to 960.85).

330. Divide: $0.62\overline{)14.5452}$. How must the decimal point be moved?

. . . .

Move the decimal point two places to the right in the denominator (0.62 becomes 62) and two places to the right in the numerator (14.5452 becomes 1454.52) so that the divisor becomes a whole number:

```
        23.46
62 ) 1454.52
     124
     214
     186
      28 5
      24 8
       3 72
       3 72
```

331. $9.8\overline{)0.49}$

. . . .

0.05

```
            0.05
98 ) 4.90
     4 90
```

332. Outline the procedure for dividing mixed decimals.

. . . .

Check page 162, Item 7.

333. What is a student's score if she answers correctly 23 out of 25 questions? Give the answer as a ratio, as a decimal fraction, and as a percent.

. . . .

ratio: $\frac{23}{25}$

The ratio of number of correct answers to number of answers is $^{23}/_{25}$.

decimal fraction: 0.92

To calculate the equivalent decimal fraction, divide:

$$\begin{array}{r} 0.92 \\ 25\overline{)23.00} \\ \underline{22\ 5} \\ 50 \\ \underline{50} \end{array}$$

percent: 92%

To calculate the score as a percent:

$$0.92 = \frac{92}{100} = 92\%$$

333a.

If you answer correctly 51 questions out of 68, what is your score as a common fraction? as a decimal? as a percent?

. . . .

$\frac{3}{4}$; 0.75; 75%

$$\frac{51}{68} = \frac{3}{4}$$

$$\begin{array}{r} 0.75 \\ 4\overline{)3.00} \end{array}$$

$$0.75 = \frac{75}{100} = 75\%$$

---

334. A 3-inch bandage is to be divided into 8 equal bandages. What is the length, in decimal form, of each small bandage? (First estimate.)

. . . .

0.375 inch

To estimate, first reason that a 4-inch bandage would be divided into 8 equal parts of $\frac{1}{2}$ *inch each. A 3-inch bandage would have 8 smaller parts. To calculate the exact size of the little bandages, divide 3 by 8:*

$$\begin{array}{r} 0.375 \\ 8\overline{)3.000} \end{array}$$

Notice that $0.375 = \frac{375}{1000} = \frac{3}{8}$ *(dividing numerator and denominator by 125) The bandage is 0.375 inch, almost* $\frac{1}{2}$ *inch.*

334a.

Use division to change the following fractions to decimal fractions: $\dfrac{15}{16}$; $\dfrac{7}{64}$.

. . . .

$$\dfrac{0.9375}{16\,\overline{)\,15.0000}}\,;\;\dfrac{0.109375}{64\,\overline{)\,7.000000}}$$

---

335. Solve for x: $3 : x = 0.25 : 8$.

. . . .

$x = 96$

$$\dfrac{3}{x} = \dfrac{0.25}{8}$$

$0.25x = 24$

$$x = \dfrac{24}{0.25}$$

$$0.25\,\overline{)\,24}$$

$$\begin{array}{r} 96 \\ 25\,\overline{)\,2400} \\ 225 \\ \hline 150 \\ 150 \\ \hline \end{array}$$

335a.

Solve for x: $0.3 : x = 0.003 : 9$.

. . . .

90

$$\dfrac{0.3}{x} = \dfrac{0.003}{.9}$$

$0.003x = 0.27$

$$x = \dfrac{0.27}{0.003}$$

$$0.003\,\overline{)\,0.27}$$

$$\begin{array}{r} 90 \\ 3\,\overline{)\,270} \end{array}$$

Rounding

336. A student answered 115 questions of the 137 given on the achievement test. What was her score? Round your answer to two decimal places.

. . . .

0.84

Carry out the division to one extra place:

$$
\begin{array}{r}
0.839 \\
137\overline{)115.000} \\
109\ 6 \\
\hline
5\ 40 \\
4\ 11 \\
\hline
1\ 290
\end{array}
$$

0.839 is between 0.830 and 0.840 and is closer to 0.840. The score would be given as 0.84.

336a.

Round the following scores to 2 decimal places:

(a) 0.913

(b) 0.917

. . . .

(a) 0.913 is greater than 0.910 and less than 0.920, but it is closer to 0.910; therefore 0.913 is rounded to 0.91.

(b) 0.917 is greater than 0.910 and less than 0.920, but it is closer to 0.920. Therefore 0.917 is rounded to 0.92.

---

337. Change $\frac{2}{35}$ to a decimal fraction, rounding the result to:

(a) 1 decimal place

(b) 2 decimal places

(c) 3 decimal places

In each case carry out the computation to *1 place more* than the place needed and round.

. . . .

(a)　　0.05　　　　　　　　　　*(a) Round 0.05²⁵⁄₃₅ to .1*

　　35) 2.00

　　　　1 75

　　　　　25

(b)　　0.057　　　　　　　　　　*(b) Round 0.057 to .06*

　　35) 2.000

　　　　1 75

　　　　　250

　　　　　245

　　　　　　5

(c)　　0.0571　　　　　　　　　*(c) Round 0.0571 to 0.057*

　　35) 2.0000

　　　　1 75

　　　　　250

　　　　　245

　　　　　　50

　　　　　　35

　　　　　　15

337a.

Change $\frac{1}{15}$ to a decimal fraction, rounding the result to:

(a) 1 decimal place

(b) 2 decimal places

(c) 3 decimal places

In each case carry out the computation to 1 place more than the place needed and round.

. . . .

(a)　　0.06　　　　　　　　　　*(a) Round 0.06 to 0.1*

　　15) 1.00

　　　　　90

　　　　　10

(b)　　0.066　　　　　　　　　*(b) Round 0.066 to 0.07*

　　15) 1.000

　　　　　90

　　　　　100

　　　　　 90

(c)　　0.0666　　　　　　　　*(c) Round 0.0666 to 0.067*

　　15) 1.0000

　　　　　90

　　　　　100

　　　　　 90

　　　　　100

　　　　　 90

SUMMARY

1. A decimal fraction is equivalent to a proper fraction with 10, 100, 1000, etc., in the denominator.

2. The number of decimal places in a decimal fraction corresponds to the number of zeros in the denominator of the equivalent proper fraction.

   Examples: $\dfrac{76}{100}$ = 0.76; two zeros in 100 and two decimal places

   0.017 = $\dfrac{17}{1000}$; three decimal places, and three zeros in 1000

3. If zeros are inserted directly to the right of the decimal point in a decimal fraction, the value of the fraction is decreased; if zeros are inserted to the right of the last digit in a decimal fraction, the value of the fraction is unchanged.

   Examples: 0.17 is greater than 0.017, 0.0017, etc.

   0.17 is equal to 0.170, 0.1700, etc.

4. To add or subtract mixed decimals, add zeros where appropriate (without changing value) so that all numbers have the same number of decimal places. Do the same for size comparisons.

   Example: To add 4.012, 0.3, 10.10172, 0.0099:

4.01200	
0.30000	The smallest value is seen to be
10.10172	0.00990.
0.00990	

5. To multiply by 10, 100, 1000, etc., move the decimal point one, two, three, etc., places to the right; to divide by 10, 100, 1000, etc., move the decimal point one, two, three, etc., places to the left. The number of places is determined by the number of zeros in 10, 100, 1000, etc.

   Examples: 0.017 × 10 = 0.17,   0.3 × 100 = 30,   0.1017 × 1000 = 101.7

6. The product of mixed decimals has the same number of decimal places as the sum of the decimal places in the original numbers.

   Example: 71.356   3 decimal places

   × 0.01   +2 decimal places

   0.71356   5 decimal places

7. When dividing, move the decimal points in the numerator and denominator an equal number of places to the right, so that the denominator becomes a whole number.

   Example: $0.352\overline{)7.2}$ $\longrightarrow$ $352.\overline{)7200.}$

8. Division should be carried out to one more place than the number of decimal places that are to appear in the rounded answer.

   Example: Find $7.2 \div 0.352$ and round to *two* decimal places:

   $$0.352\overline{)7.2} \quad \longrightarrow \quad 352\overline{)7200} \quad \longrightarrow \quad 352\overline{)7200.000}$$

   $$\uparrow$$

   three decimal places

EXERCISES FOR EXTRA PRACTICE

1. Write as mixed numbers or proper fractions.

   (a) 3.24   (b) 41.02   (c) 1.2003   (d) 7.40

   (e) 7.04   (f) 70.4   (g) 2.7   (h) 0.27

   (i) 0.00027

2. Write as decimal fractions or mixed decimals.

   (a) $\dfrac{3}{10}$ (b) $\dfrac{77}{100}$ (c) $5\dfrac{3}{1000}$ (d) $\dfrac{3}{50}$

   (e) $\dfrac{1}{200}$ (f) $\dfrac{7}{20}$ (g) $\dfrac{107}{100}$ (h) forty-two hundredths

   (i) forty and two hundredths   (j) 62%   (k) $8\dfrac{1}{2}\%$ (l) 3.02%

3. In each of the following cases, choose the decimal fraction representing the larger value.

   (a) 0.01, 0.0009   (b) 0.919, 0.9

   (c) 0.23, 0.2003   (d) 0.007, 0.06

   (e) 0.1734, 0.01744   (f) 0.101095, 0.10111

4. Add and round to two decimal places.

   (a) 7.01 + 2.0009 + 1.234   (b) 0.919 + 4.9 + 0.03

   (c) 0.007 + 1.06 + 2.1011   (d) 3.03 + 2.1 + 0.0003

   (e) 0.1 + 2.005 + 0.3201   (f) 32.46 + 3.012

5. Subtract.

   (a) 5.004 − 4.2   (b) 54.68 − 5.004   (c) 100 − 0.059

6. Multiply.

   (a) 0.059 by 10   (b) 9.02 by 100   (c) 0.10111 by 1000

   (d) 7.057 by 23   (e) 1.035 by 7.2   (f) 0.41 by 0.3

7. Divide, using the numbers given in Exercise 6, and round to four decimal places.

8. Change to percents.

   (a) 0.34   (b) 0.034   (c) 3.40   (d) 1.253

   (e) 0.0012   (f) 0.2

. . . .

Answers

1. (a) $3\frac{6}{25}$ (b) $41\frac{1}{50}$ (c) $1\frac{2,003}{10,000}$ (d) $7\frac{2}{5}$

   (e) $7\frac{1}{25}$ (f) $70\frac{2}{5}$ (g) $2\frac{7}{10}$ (h) $\frac{27}{100}$

   (i) $\frac{27}{100,000}$

2. (a) 0.3   (b) 0.77   (c) 5.003   (d) 0.06

   (e) 0.005   (f) 0.35   (g) 1.07   (h) 0.42

   (i) 40.02   (j) 0.62   (k) 0.085   (l) 0.0302

3. (a) 0.0100   (b) 0.919   (c) 0.2300   (d) 0.060

   (e) 0.17340   (f) 0.101110

4. (a) 10.24   (b) 5.85   (c) 3.17   (d) 5.13

   (e) 2.43   (f) 35.47

5. (a) 0.804   (b) 49.676   (c) 99.941

6. (a) 0.59   (b) 902   (c) 101.11   (d) 162.311

   (e) 7.452   (f) 0.123

7. (a) 0.0059   (b) 0.0902   (c) 0.0001   (d) 0.3068

   (e) 0.1438   (f) 1.3667

8. (a) 34%   (b) 3.4%   (c) 340%   (d) 125.3%

   (e) 0.12%   (f) 20%

INVENTORY

The set of exercises below will show you whether you are already an expert or whether you need a little more practice. If you do need more practice, the numbers next to the answers will direct you to the particular frames that should receive your special attention.

1. Write in words 700.06.

2. Write as a mixed number 263.067.

3. Use decimal notation:
   (a) two hundred and three hundredths.
   (b) two hundred three thousandths.

4. Arrange in order of size (smallest first):   100.001, 0.1001, 0.0101, 1.010.

5. Add the above numbers.

6. Subtract 2.357 from 23.57.

7. Multiply 1.89 × 1000; divide 64.8 by 1000.

8. Multiply 73 by 0.023.

9. Divide 0.0616 by 4.

10. Divide 18 by 4 and express the answer as a mixed decimal.

11. Divide 0.32 by 1.6.

12. Express $\frac{3}{7}$ as a 2-place decimal fraction.

13. Change to decimals: 12%, 9.2%, 0.023%.

14. Change to percents: 2.45, 0.102, 0.002.

. . . .

Answers

1. Seven hundred and six hundredths (Frames 289—291)

2. $263^{67}/_{1000}$ (Frame 289)

3. (a) 200.03; (b) 0.203 (Frames 261, 289)

4. 0.0101, 0.1001, 1.010, 100.001 (Frames 278, 281, 289)

5. 101.1212 (Frames 282—295)

6. 21.213 (Frames 282—295)

7. 1890.0 (Frames 296—301); 0.0648 (Frames 302—310)

8. 1.679 (Frames 317—331)

9. 0.0154 (Frames 331—333)

10. 4.5 (Frames 331—333)

11. 0.2 (Frames 331—333)

12. 0.43 (Frames 333—335)

13. 0.12, 0.092, 0.00023 (Frames 311—313)

14. 245%, 10.2%, 0.2% (Frames 314—316)

If you have no incorrect answers, proceed to Section 7. Otherwise, study the relevant frames and then go back to the Proficiency Gauge on page 127.

SYSTEMS OF MEASUREMENT
THE APOTHECARIES' SYSTEM

The grave responsibility of measuring drugs to prepare or check dosages frequently falls on the nurse. In the United States, there are two systems of measurement: the apothecaries' system and the metric system. Both of these systems are still in common use, although the metric system is preferred and is growing in importance.

In carrying out the physician's orders, it is clear that the nurse must be able to weigh and measure, and convert from one system of measurement to the other. She must be able to calculate with Roman numerals, which are used with the apothecaries' system of weights and measures, as well as with decimal numbers, which are used with the metric system.

After completion of this section, the student should be able to:

1. Name the units of weight and liquid capacity in the apothecaries' system.

2. Express a given measurement in terms of any of the units.

3. Write out measurements in symbols appropriate for a prescription.

PROFICIENCY GAUGE

1. What is the basic unit of weight in the apothecaries' system?

2. What is the basic unit of liquid (or fluid) capacity in the apothecaries' system?

3. Find the number of grains in gr. xxvii, using Arabic numerals.

4. Write in symbols appropriate for a prescription: 77 grains, 24 grains, 98 grains.

5. Write in symbols: 2 pounds, 5 ounces, $3\frac{1}{2}$ drams; also 2 gallons, 1 quart, 1 pint, 4 fluidounces, 2 fluidrams, and $3\frac{1}{2}$ minims.

6. What part of a dram is gr. xv? What part of a pint is f℥ lxiv?

. . . .

Answers

1. the grain	4. gr. lxxvii, gr. xxiv, gr. xcviii
2. the minim	5. lb. ii, ℥v, ℈iiiss, Cii, qt. i, Oi, ℥iv, f℈ii, ℳiiiss
3. 27	6. ¼, ½

The apothecaries' system is a very old system of measurement, originating in Greece, Rome, and France. It was in use in England in the 17th century and spread to the New World with the English colonists. We will first consider the system of weights and later turn our attention to measures of capacity.

Basic Unit of Weight

338. Like most ancient systems of measurement, the apothecaries' system of weights is based on a familiar farm object: a *grain* of wheat. At one time, such a unit of weight was quite unreliable inasmuch as grains of wheat grew in many different sizes. Today, however, the *grain* is fixed according to international standards; it is defined in relation to a cubic inch of distilled water at its greatest density with 30 inches of barometric pressure. If we were to measure the weight of the familiar pound loaf of bread according to the apothecaries' system, we would find that its weight was about 7000 grains. The small-family loaf (½ pound) would weigh about _____ .

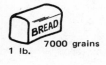

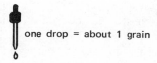

one drop = about 1 grain

. . . .

3500 grains

339. One day you may have to carry out a doctor's order to dissolve one-quarter grain of morphine sulfate in a solution. You may see it written in symbols on a prescription, gr. ¼. How would you expect to see one-third grain written?

. . . .

gr. $\frac{1}{3}$

340. Write in symbols appropriate for a prescription: one-tenth grain.

. . . .

gr. $\frac{1}{10}$

341. What is wrong with the following symbols for one-fifth grain? $\frac{1}{5}$ gr.

. . . .

It should be gr. $\frac{1}{5}$.

---

342. A tablet contains one grain of phenobarbital. If the tablet is dissolved and then administered in 4 equal portions, each portion contains _____ of phenobarbital. (Use symbols.)

. . . .

gr. $\dfrac{1}{4}$

Roman Numerals

---

343. Fractional parts of a grain are expressed in Arabic numerals: gr. $\frac{1}{4}$, gr. $\frac{1}{8}$, gr. $\frac{1}{2}$, etc., but one or more grains require the use of lowercase Roman numerals. For instance, the usual aspirin tablet contains gr. v of aspirin, since _____ is the Roman numeral for 5.

. . . .

v

---

344. If you have forgotten how to use Roman numerals go right on to Frame 345. If you are very familiar with Roman numerals, fill in the following tables. If you have no errors, skip to Frame 364.

Roman	Arabic
xii	12
	53
	11
	7
	100
vi	
ii	
iv	

Roman	Arabic
ix	
xl	
xix	
xc	
xcix	
	96
	58
	59

. . . .

Roman	Arabic
liii	53
xi	11
vii	7
c	100
vi	6
ii	2
iv	4

Roman	Arabic
ix	9
xl	40
xix	19
xc	90
xcix	99
xcvi	96
lviii	58
lix	59

345. A table of Roman numerals will be found in the Appendix.   Do *not* refer to the Appendix, however, for the following exercises. The Roman numerals most commonly used in prescriptions are i, v, x, l, c. Study the following:

i   is the Roman numeral for 1—think of one person.

v   is the Roman numeral for 5—some historians think it represented an outstretched hand to the Romans.

x   is the Roman numeral for 10—it represented two hands one up and one down.

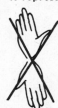

l   is the Roman numeral for 50—middle life!

c   is the Roman numeral for 100—think of 100¢ in a dollar.

Write the Roman numerals corresponding to the following Arabic numerals: 1, 5, 10, 50, 100.

. . . .

1 ⟶ i

5 ⟶ v

10 ⟶ x

50 ⟶ l

100 ⟶ c

346. Fill in the blank spaces with the corresponding Arabic numerals:

i	l	x	c	v

. . . .

    1 50 10 100 5

347. The symbol for two grains is gr. ii. The symbol for three grains is _____ .

. . . .

gr. iii

348. Write in words: gr. vi.

. . . .

six grains

349. Write in symbols: eight grains.

. . . .

gr. viii

350. Given that the symbol for 10 grains is gr. x, write the symbols for 11, 12, and 13 grains.

. . . .

gr. xi, gr. xii, gr. xiii

351. A certain tablet contains 26 grains of salt. How many grains in two such tablets? (Use symbols.)

. . . .

gr. lii

352. Fill in the blank spaces with the corresponding Roman or Arabic numerals:

Roman	xii		vi		ii		
Arabic	12	53		11		7	100

. . . .

Roman: liii, xi, vii, c;   Arabic: 6, 2

353. Fill in the blank spaces with the corresponding Roman or Arabic numerals:

Roman	x	xx	
Arabic	10		30

. . . .

Roman: xxx;   Arabic: 20

354. Match each Roman numeral on the left with the corresponding Arabic numeral on the right:

xv   32
xvi   66
xxi   17
xvii   15
xxxvi   21
xxxii   36
lxvi   16

. . . .

xv   15
xvi   16
xxi   21
xvii   17
xxxvi   36
xxxii   32
lxvi   66

355. The values of all the Roman numerals in the preceding exercises have been found by (adding/subtracting) the numbers represented by the numerals. For example: lxxvi = 50 + 10 + 10 + 5 + 1 + 1 = 77. In every case, the (greater/smaller) numbers are written first.

. . . .

adding; greater

---

356. Usually the smaller Roman numbers *follow* the larger; whenever a smaller number *follows* a larger, the numbers are *added*. If the smaller number should *precede* the larger, the smaller must be (added/subtracted).

. . . .

subtracted

---

357. Complete the table with the corresponding Arabic numerals:

iv	ix	xl	xix	xc	xcix
4		40		90	

. . . .

9, 19, 99

---

358. The principle of subtraction is used only in cases where 4 and 9 are involved.

gr. iv   =   4 grains

gr. ix   =   9 grains

gr. xl   = 40 grains

gr. xcix = 99 grains

Write the following symbols using Arabic numerals: gr. xiv, gr. xxiv, gr. xlix, gr. lxiv, gr. xciv

. . . .

14, 24, 49, 64, 94 grains

359. Write in Roman numerals: 96.

. . . .

xcvi

360. Write 58 and 59 in Roman numerals.

. . . .

lviii, lix

361. Choose the correct answer or answers. The principle of subtraction is used in writing the following number(s) in Roman numerals: 58 only, 59 only, 58 and 59.

. . . .

59 only

362. Which is greater: cx or xc?

. . . .

cx

363. If a dose of medicine weighs gr. xiv, two such doses will weigh _____ . (Use symbols.)

. . . .

gr. xxviii

Other Units of Weight

364. The _____ is the fundamental unit of weight in the apothecaries' system. Larger units of weight in the same system are the *dram*, the *ounce*, and the *pound*. The appropriate symbols are given on the next page. Copy the words with their symbols. Practice the symbol for each unit of weight several times.

dram: ℥ (weight of about 1 scant teaspoonful of water)

ounce: ℥ (weight of about 2 scant tablespoonsful of water)

pound: lb.

The abbreviation for pound comes from the Latin word for pound, *libra*.   The apothecary ounce and pound come from the Troy system of measurement, originating in Troyes, France, in the 14th century.

. . . .

grain

---

365.   Write the following sentence as an equation using symbols: Sixty grains equals one dram.

. . . .

gr. lx = ℥ i

For Frames 366–375 refer to Table A in the Appendix.

---

366.   How many grains are there in ℥ $\frac{1}{3}$?   (Use symbols.)

. . . .

gr. xx

---

367.   How many grains in ℥ ii?

. . . .

120 or gr. cxx

---

368. A doctor's prescription calls for gr. xv of a certain drug. The drug comes in packets of ℨi. What part of the packet would be used?

. . . .

$\dfrac{1}{4}$ $\dfrac{15}{60} = \dfrac{1}{4}$

369. A dosage of gr. lxxv is the equivalent of a dosage of ℨ _____ and gr. _____ .

. . . .

ℨi and gr. xv

370. The symbol for one-half dram is ℨ½. However if ½ is used in conjunction with a whole number, a special symbol is used: ss (from the Latin, *semis*, meaning half). Thus, one and one-half drams is written ℨiss. The symbols for two and one-half drams are _____ .

. . . .

ℨiiss

371. Write in words: ℨ viiss.

. . . .

seven and one-half drams

372. Find the number of grains in an ounce.

. . . .

480

373. Which is heavier, a pound of drugs or a pound of bread?

. . . .

A pound of bread is heavier; it weighs 16 ounces, avoirdupois weight. This is equivalent to about 15 ounces in apothecary weight.

A pound of drugs weighs only 12 ounces, apothecary weight. People are usually more familiar with avoirdupois weight, in which 16 ounces = 1 pound. The latter is used for weighing all particles except drugs, gold, silver, and precious stones.

374. Since a drop of water weighs about one grain, the following code (Grain Drop 60-8-12) may help you remember the apothecary units of weight.

G R A I N	D R	O	P	60	8	12
(basic unit: gr.)	dram ʒ	o u n c e ʒ	p o u n d lb.	60 grains to a dram	8 d r a m s to an o u n c e	12 ounces to a pound

Find the number of drams in 3 pounds. Write your answer in symbols.

. . . .

ʒ cclxxxviii

12 ounces =	1 pound
36 ounces =	3 pounds
8 drams =	1 ounce
288 drams =	36 ounces

375. Find the number of grains in ʒ iiiss. Write the answer in symbols.

. . . .

gr. ccx

$x\ grains = 3\frac{1}{2}\ drams$

$60\ grains = 1\ dram$

$$\frac{x}{60} = \frac{3\frac{1}{2}}{1}$$

$$x = 3\frac{1}{2} \times 60$$

$$x = \frac{7}{2_1} \times \cancel{60}^{30} = 210\ grains$$

Units of Fluid Capacity

376. The apothecaries' system of *weight* is based on the _____ ; the apothecaries' system of fluid *capacity* is based on the *minim*. The minim is a quantity
of water that weighs approximately one grain. Thus two minims of water would
weigh approximately _____ . (Use symbols.)

. . . .

grain; gr. ii

---

377. The symbol for minims is ♏. Write the expression for 24 minims as it should be
written in a prescription.

. . . .

♏ xxiv

---

378. The _____ is the basic unit of fluid capacity in the apothecaries' system.
Larger units are the fluidram, the fluid ounce, the pint, the quart, and the gallon.
The appropriate symbols are given below. Copy the words with their symbols.
Practice the symbols for each unit several times.

minims: ♏

fluidram: f ʒ   (about 1 scant teaspoonful)

fluid ounce: f ℥   (about 2 tablespoonsful)

pint: pt. or O (about 2 glasses)

quart: at.   (about 4 glasses)

gallon: gal. or C

The abbreviation for pint, O, comes from the Latin word *octavius* meaning an eighth (of a gallon); the symbol for gallon, C, is from the Latin word *congius*, meaning a container with capacity 1 gallon.

. . . .

minim

For Frames 379—388 refer to Table B in the Appendix.

---

379. Rewrite the following sentence using symbols only: Sixteen fluid ounces equal 1 pint.

. . . .

f ℥ xvi = pt. i

---

380. Since the volume of a drop of water is about 1 minim, the following code (min-drop 60-8-16-2-4) may help you remember the apothecary units of fluid capacity.

M I N	D R	O	P	60	8	16	2	4
minim ♏	flui-dram f ʒ	fluid ounce f ℥	pint pt. or O	60 minims in a flui-dram	8 flui-drams in a fluid ounce	16 fluid ounces in a pint	2 pints in a quart	4 quarts in a gallon

About how much do 60 minims of water weigh?

. . . .

about 60 grains or 1 dram

---

381. How many fluidrams in f ℥ vi? (Use symbols only.)

. . . .

f ℥ vi = f ʒ xlviii

382. How many fluid ounces in pt. $\frac{1}{4}$? (Use symbols only.)

. . . .

pt. $\frac{1}{4}$ = f ℥ iv

---

383. A doctor's prescription calls for ℔ xv of a certain drug. The drug comes in vials of f ℥ i. What part of the vial should be used?

. . . .

$\frac{1}{4}$

60 minims = 1 fluidram
15 minims = x fluidrams

$$\frac{x}{1} = \frac{15}{60} = \frac{1}{4}$$

15 minims = $\frac{1}{4}$ fluidram

---

384. A dosage of ℔ lxvss is the equivalent of a dosage of f ℥ _____ and ℔ _____ .

. . . .

f ℥ i; ℔ vss

$65\frac{1}{2}$ minims = 60 minims + $5\frac{1}{2}$ minims = 1 fluidram + $5\frac{1}{2}$ minims

---

385. Find the number of minims in a fluid ounce.

. . . .

480 minims

8 fluidrams = 1 fluid ounce
x minims   = 8 fluidrams
60 minims   = 1 fluidram

$$\frac{x}{60} = \frac{8}{1}$$

$$x = 480$$

386. Find the number of ounces of holiday drink in a punch bowl filled with eggnog if 3 quarts of dairy eggnog have been mixed with 24 ounces of rum and 1½ pints of whipped cream.

. . . .

144

1 quart = 2 pints
3 quarts = 6 pints
3 quarts + 1½ pints = 7½ pints
1 pint   = 16 ounces
7½ pints = 16 × 7½ = 120 ounces
120 + 24 = 144

387. Complete:

(a) f ℥ iiss = _____ minims.

(b) f ℥ iss = f ℥ _____ .

(c) Two gallons contain _____ pints.

. . . .

(a) 150

(b) xii

(c) 16

388. Compare the table of fluid capacity with the table of fluid weights. Which relationships are similar?

. . . .

gr. lx = ℈ i   and   ♏ lx = f ℥ i;
℈ viii = ℥ i   and   f ℈ viii = f ℥ i

SUMMARY

1. Using the apothecaries' system, a drop of water weighs about 1 grain. There are 60 grains in a dram, 8 drams in an ounce, 12 ounces to a pound. In symbols:

   gr. lx = ℨ i

   ℨ viii = ℥ i

   ℥ xii = lb. i

   See Table A in the Appendix.

   Example: To find the number of grains in ℨ $\frac{1}{3}$, multiply $\frac{1}{3}$ by 60. There are gr. xx in ℨ $\frac{1}{3}$.

2. Using the apothecaries' system, the volume of a drop of water is about 1 minim. There are 60 minims in a fluidram, 8 drams in a fluid ounce, 16 ounces in a pint, 2 pints in a quart, 4 quarts in a gallon. In symbols:

   ♏ lx = f ℨ i

   f ℨ viii = f ℥ i

   f ℥ xvi = pt. i

   pt. ii = qt. i

   qt. iv = gal. i

   See Table B in the Appendix.

EXERCISES FOR EXTRA PRACTICE

1. f ℥ xxiv = f ℥ _____

2. ℥ xxxii = ℥ _____

3. f ℥ viii = pt. _____

4. ℥ iiss = gr. _____

5. pt. xvi = gal. _____

6. pt. ii = f ℥ _____

7. gr. xxx = ℥ _____

8. ℥ ii = ℥ _____

9. ♍ xv = f ℥ _____

10. f ℥ iss =- f ℥ _____

. . . .

Answers

1. iii

2. iv

3. $\frac{1}{2}$

4. cl

5. ii

6. xxxii

7. $\frac{1}{2}$

8. xvi

9. $\frac{1}{4}$

10. xii

INVENTORY

Answer the following questions. If you have errors, study the relevant frames and then go back to the Proficiency Gauge on page 167.

1. What is the basic unit of weight in the apothecaries' system?

2. What is the basic unit of fluid capacity in the apothecaries' system?

3. Find the number of grains in gr. lxii.

4. Write in symbols appropriate for a prescription: 36 grains, 45 grains, 89 grains.

5. Write in symbols: 2 pounds, 5 ounces, $3\frac{1}{2}$ drams.

6. Write in symbols: 2 gallons, 1 quart, 1 pint, 4 fluid ounces, 2 fluidrams, and $3\frac{1}{2}$ minims.

7. What part of a dram is gr. xx?

8. What part of a fluid ounce is ℞ xxx?

. . . .

Answers

1. the grain (Frame 338)

2. the minim (Frame 376)

3. 62 (Frames 339–362)

4. gr. xxxvi, gr. xlv, gr. lxxxix (Frames 339–362)

5. lb. ii, ℥ v, ʒ iiiss (Frames 340–388)

6. Cii, qt., i, pt. i, f ℥ iv, f ʒ ii, ℞ iiiss (Frames 367–388)

7. $\frac{1}{3}$ (Frame 368)

8. $\frac{1}{16}$ (Frames 380–387)

SYSTEMS OF MEASUREMENT
THE METRIC SYSTEM

After completion of this section, the student should be able to:

1. Name the units of length, weight, and liquid capacity in the metric system.

2. Express a given measurement in terms of any of the units.

3. Convert from one system of measurements to the other.

PROFICIENCY GAUGE

1. 38 mg.   = _____ Gm.

2. 5100 mg. = _____ Gm.

3. 0.9 Gm.   = _____ mg.

4. 0.52 L.   = _____ ml.

5. 27 ml.   = _____ L.

6. 0.3 ml.   = _____ L.

7. ℔ xii   = _____ ml.

8. gr. $\frac{1}{8}$ = _____ mg.

9. ℨ xxxii   = _____ Gm.

10. f ℥ xii   = _____ cc.

. . . .

Answers

1. 0.038

2. 5.1

3. 900

4. 520

5. 0.027

6. 0.0003

7. 0.7

8. 7.5

9. 128

10. 360

Units of Length

389. In the United States, there are two systems commonly used for compounding medicines both for weights and for fluid capacity: the metric system as well as the apothecaries' system. Which system is the older system?

. . . .

the apothecaries' system

---

390. The apothecaries' system was already an old system in the 17th century when it was carried to the New World by the English colonists. The metric system, on the other hand, did not come into use until its invention in France at the end of the 18th century. Since these two systems, the _____ system and the _____ system, are used interchangeably in the United States for weighing and measuring drugs, it is necessary for the nurse to be familiar with both.

. . . .

metric; apothecaries'

---

391. The metric system is named for its basic unit of length, the meter. The meter is approximately 3 inches (shorter/longer) than the yard.

		centimeters			METER					
2 3	10	20	30	40	50	60	70	80	90	100

	YARD	
1 inch	1 foot	

. . . .

longer

---

392. Thus the meter is approximately _____ feet.

. . . .

3.3 or $3\frac{1}{3}$

393. Would a man of height 2 meters be likely to be found on a basketball court?

. . . .

Quite possibly since he would be about 6 ft., 7 in. tall.

394. The most common subdivisions of the meter are the centimeter ($\frac{1}{100}$ m.) and the millimeter ($\frac{1}{1000}$ m.). In symbols:

   100 cm. = 1 m.

   1000 mm. = 1 m.

   How many millimeters are there in a centimeter?

. . . .

10 mm. = 1 cm. For each centimeter there are 10 times as many millimeters in a meter.

395. In a beauty contest, one young woman gave her measurements as 36–24–36. What would the equivalent vital statistics be under the metric system? (Use the diagram in Frame 391 to compare inches with centimeters.)

. . . .

90 – 60 – 90 $2\frac{1}{2}$ cm. = 1 in. (approximately)

$36 \times 2\frac{1}{2} = 90; \quad 24 \times 2\frac{1}{2} = 60$

Units of Liquid Capacity

396. In addition to measures of length, the metric system includes measures of liquid capacity (based on the liter), and weights (based on the gram). The nurse is primarily interested in measures of <u>li</u>quid capacity (based on the li _____) and weights (based on the _____).

. . . .

liter; gram

397. The liter is slightly more than a quart; actually the _____ is equal to 1.06 quart.

. . . .

1 liter   MILK   MILK   1 quart

liter

---

398. A child who drinks 4 liters of milk per week is drinking a little (more/less) than 4 quarts of milk per week.

. . . .

more

---

399. The abbreviation for liter is L. If a container is said to have 4 L. of water, the quantity of water in the container is 4 _____ .

. . . .

liters

---

400. Seven liters may be written in abbreviated form as 7 _____ .

. . . .

L.

---

401. The liter is often subdivided for convenience into 1000 parts. Each subdivision is called a milliliter. Thus $\frac{1}{1000}$ of a liter is a _____ .

. . . .

MILK 1 LITER   1000 milliliters

milliliter

---

402. Milliliter means $\frac{1}{1000}$ of a liter, just as millimeter means $\frac{1}{1000}$ of a meter, and milligram means $\frac{1}{1000}$ of a gram. The part of the word milliliter that means $\frac{1}{1000}$ is _____ .

. . . .

milli

---

403. 1000 milliliters are the equivalent of 1 _____ .

. . . .

liter

---

404. A liter contains _____ milliliters.

. . . .

1000

---

405. A container of capacity of 1 liter can hold 1000 _____ .

. . . .

milliliters

---

406. The Soviet Union announced that it is developing a 3-liter "bath," (pieces of cheesecloth soaked with a special liquid) for astronauts to use in space. How many milliliters would this be?

. . . .

3000

406a.

A container holding two liters of liquid holds _____ milliliters.

. . . .

2000

---

407. The abbreviation for milliliter is ml. Therefore 2 L. = _____ ml.

. . . .

2000

---

408. To change from liters to milliliters, multiply the number of liters by _____ .

. . . .

1000

409. How many milliliters are there in 5 liters?

. . . .

5000

410. In changing 5 liters to 5000 milliliters, you (multiplied/divided) by (100/1000).

. . . .

multiplied; 1000

411. In changing 2 L. to 2000 ml., we must _____ 2 by _____ .

. . . .

multiply; 1000

412. Change 4 L. to ml. The number of milliliters is (greater/less) than the number of liters.

. . . .

4000; greater

413. 2 L. = 2000 ml.
    3 L. = 3000 ml.
    4 L. = 4000 ml.

Each number on the left has been _____ by 1000 to get the number on the right. In multiplying by 1000, the decimal place is moved _____ places to the _____ .

. . . .

multiplied; three; right

414. To change 3.91 L. to ml., _____ 3.91 by 1000. Thus 3.91 L. = _____ ml.

. . . .

multiply; 3910

414a.

52.3 liters are equivalent to _____ milliliters.

. . . .

52,300

415. A container holding 0.032 L. holds _____ ml.

. . . .

32

416. 9000 ml. = _____ L.

. . . .

9

417. Which is bigger, a liter or a milliliter? If a container holds a certain number of liters, will it hold fewer or more milliliters?

. . . .

liter; more

418. In expressing a given capacity in liters or milliliters, the number of milliliters is (greater/less) than the given number of liters?

. . . .

greater

419. In changing the expressed measure of a given capacity from milliliters to liters, the number of liters will be (less/greater) than the given number of milliliters?

. . . .

less

420. 5000 ml. = _____ L.   6000 ml. = _____ L.

. . . .

5; 6

421. To change from milliliters to liters, divide the number of milliliters by _____.

. . . .

1000

422. 3000 ml. = 3 L. To change from 3000 ml. to 3 L., _____ 3000 by _____ . This is equivalent to moving the decimal point _____ places to the _____ .

. . . .

divide by 1000; three; left

423. Moving the decimal point to the _____ is equivalent to dividing; the resulting number is (less/greater) than the original.

. . . .

left; less

424. To express 2956 ml. in liters, _____ 2956 by 1000.

. . . .

divide

425. 12.91 ml. = _____ L.

. . . .

0.01291

425a.

347.2 ml. = _____ L.

. . . .

0.3472

426. Which is greater, 2 L. or 400 ml.?

. . . .

2 L.

427. The liter and milliliter are used to measure _____ capacity in the
_____ system.

. . . .

liquid (or fluid); metric

428. Further useful relationships can be seen from the following diagram:

1000
Cubic
centimeters

Equals
(approximately)

1
Liter

In symbols, 1000 cc. = 1 L. (approximately) and 1 cc. = _____ ml.
approximately).

. . . .

1   *1000 cc. = 1 L.*

$$1 \ cc. = \frac{1}{1000} \ L. = 1 \ ml.$$

Units of Weight

429. The meter is a unit of length and the liter is a unit of capacity in the metric system. The *gram* is a unit of *weight* in the metric system. The unit of weight,
called the (liter/gram) is the weight of 1 ml. of water at 4° Celsius.

. . . .

gram

---

430. At 4° Celsius, 1 ml. of water weighs 1 _____ .

. . . .

gram

---

431. At 4° Celsius, 1 cc. of water weighs about 1 _____ .

. . . .

gram   *Remember that 1 cc. = 1 ml. approximately.*

---

432. The weight of 2 ml. of water at 4° Celsius is 2 _____ .

. . . .

grams

---

433. Alcohol is lighter than water. Therefore 2 ml. of alcohol at 4° Celsius weigh less
than or more than 2 grams?

. . . .

less than

433a.

1 ml. of a liquid that is heavier than 1 ml. of _____ at 4° Celsius weighs more than 1 gram.

. . . .

water

434. An ounce is about 30 times heavier than a gram. At 4° Celsius, 1 ml. of water weighs much (more/less) than an ounce.

about 30 grams

. . . .

less

435. The abbreviation for gram is Gm. Thus 2.3 Gm. = 2.3 _____ .

. . . .

grams

436. At 4° Celsius, 100 cc. of water weigh about _____ .

. . . .

100 Gm.

437. 50 ml. of water weigh about _____ .

. . . .

50 Gm.

438. The volume of 1 Gm. of water is about 1 _____ , or 1 _____ .

. . . .

1 cc.; 1 ml.

439. A liter contains 1000 milliliters. A gram contains 1000 _____ grams.

. . . .

milli

---

440. 1 Gm. = 1000 _____ .

. . . .

milligrams

---

441. The abbreviation for milligram is mg. Thus 1 Gm. = _____ mg.

1000 mg

. . . .

1000

---

442. 3 Gm. = _____ mg.

. . . .

3000

---

443. To express a given number of grams in milligrams, _____ the number of grams by 1000.

. . . .

multiply

---

444. To express 0.020 Gm. in milligrams, _____ 0.020 by _____ .
Thus 0.020 Gm. = _____ mg.

. . . .

multiply; 1000; 20

444a.

To express 4 Gm. in milligrams, _____ 4 by 1000.

. . . .

multiply

---

445. A drug weighing 0.0325 Gm. weighs _____ mg.

. . . .

32.5

---

446. A drug weighing 0.073 Gm. weighs _____ mg.

. . . .

73

---

447. Drug *A* weighs 1 Gm.; drug *B* weighs 10.2 mg. Which drug is heavier?

. . . .

A   *1 Gm. = 1000 mg.*

---

448. 4000 mg. = _____ Gm.

. . . .

4

---

449. To express a given number of milligrams in grams, _____ the number of milligrams by 1000.

. . . .

divide

450. 6000 mg. = _____ Gm.

. . . .

6

---

451. 750 mg. = _____ Gm.

. . . .

0.75

---

452. 72.34 mg. = _____ Gm.

. . . .

0.07234

---

453. A kilogram (kg.) contains 1000 Gm. The volume of a kilogram of water is about _____ cc., or _____ L.

. . . .

1000; 1

1 ml. or 1 cc. weighs 1 Gm.

1000 ml. or 1000 cc. weighs 1000 Gm.

1 L. or 1000 cc. weigh 1 kg.

---

454. If a person weighs more than 90 kg., he is not permitted to take a muleback trip into the Grand Canyon. What maximum weight in pounds is allowed? (See Table G in the Appendix.)

. . . .

198 lbs.   *90 × 2.2 = 198*

Converting From One System to the Other

455. Express ♏ xlv in the metric system. (Use Table G in the Appendix.)

. . . .

3 ml.

15 minims = 1 ml.

45 minims = 3 ml.

---

456. Express 1.2 ml. in the apothecaries' system.

. . . .

18 minims

x minims = 1.2 ml.

15 minims = 1 ml.

$$\frac{x}{15} = \frac{1.2}{1}$$

x = 15 × 1.2

x = 18

---

457. Express ♏lx in the metric system.

. . . .

♏lx = 4 ml.

15 minims = 1 ml.

60 minims = 4 ml.

---

458. Find the metric equivalent of f ʒiiss.

. . . .

f ʒiiss = 10 ml.

f ʒiiss = 2½ fluidrams or 150 minims

x ml. = 150 minims

1 ml. =   15 minims

x   =   10

---

459. Express 0.8 ml. in the apothecaries' system.

. . . .

0.8 ml. = 12 minims

0.8 ml. = x minims

1 ml. = 15 minims

$$\frac{x}{15} = \frac{0.8}{1}$$

x = 15 × 0.8 = 12

SUMMARY

1. Using the metric system, a yardstick is a little less than a meter. There are 1000 millimeters in a meter and 1000 meters in a kilometer. See Table C in the Appendix.

   Example: To find the number of millimeters in 0.56 m., multiply 0.56 by 1000. There are 560 mm. in 0.56 m.

2. Using the metric system, a liquid quart is a little less than a liter and weighs about a kilogram. There are 1000 ml. in 1 L., 1000 mg. in 1 Gm., and 1000 Gm. in 1 kg. See Tables D and E in the Appendix.

   Example: To compare weights of 0.06 Gm. and 48 mg., we change 0.06 Gm. to 60 mg. by multiplying 0.06 × 1000 and note that 60 mg. is greater than 48 mg. Thus 0.06 Gm. is greater than 48 mg.

3. It is important for the nurse to be able to switch from one system to another. Table G in the Appendix gives commonly used approximate equivalents.

   Example: If medication is ordered in doses of 5 ml., the number of fluid ounces needed for 12 doses would be found as follows:

$$\frac{\text{fluid ounces needed}}{1 \text{ fluid ounce}} = \frac{\text{ml. needed}}{\text{ml. in 1 fluid ounce}}$$

$$\frac{x}{1} = \frac{12 \times 5}{30}$$

$$x = 2.$$

EXERCISES FOR EXTRA PRACTICE

1. (a) 530 mg. = _____ Gm.   (b) 0.0003 Gm. = _____ mg.

   (c) 24 mg = _____ Gm.   (d) _____ mg. = 0.087 Gm.

   (e) 16 mg. = _____ Gm.   (f) 0.064 Gm. = _____ mg.

   (g) 1500 mg. = _____ Gm.   (h) _____ mg. = 0.4 Gm.

   (i) 0.35 L. = _____ ml.   (j) 75 ml. = _____ L.

   (k) 0.1 Gm. = _____ mg.   (l) 0.2 ml. = _____ L.

2. (a) 15 cc. = f ℥ _____   (b) 0.6 mg. = gr. _____

   (c) _____ ml. = f ℨ iiss.   (d) ℨ xvi = _____ Gm.

   (e) 360 cc. = f ℥ _____   (f) 90 Gm. = ℨ _____

   (g) gr $\frac{1}{5}$ = _____ mg.   (h) f ℥ xvi = _____ ml.

   (i) _____ Gm. = gr. v   (j) f ℨ xvi = _____ L.

   (k) 20 ml. = f ℨ _____   (l) 15 mg. = gr. _____

. . . .

Answers

1. (a) 0.53   (b) 0.3   (c) 0.024   (d) 87

   (e) 0.016   (f) 64   (g) 1.5   (h) 400

   (i) 350   (j) 0.075   (k) 100   (l) 0.0002

2. (a) ss   (b) $\frac{1}{100}$ (c) 10   (d) 64

   (e) xii   (f) xxiv   (g) 12   (h) 480

   (i) 0.3   (j) 0.064   (k) v   (l) gr. $\frac{1}{4}$

INVENTORY

1. 36 mg. = _____ Gm.

2. _____ mg. = 0.025 Gm.

3. 4500 mg. = _____ Gm.

4. 320 mg. = _____ Gm.

5. 0.0001 Gm. = _____ mg.

6. 0.25 L. = _____ ml.

7. 50 ml. = _____ L.

8. ℳ _____ = 1.5 ml.

9. gr. _____ = 0.6 Gm.

10. f ℥ iss = _____ c.c.

. . . .

Answers

1. 0.036 (Frames 448—452)

2. 25 (Frames 439—446)

3. 4.5 (Frames 448—452)

4. 0.32 (Frames 000—000)

5. 0.1 (Frames 439—446)

6. 250 (Frames 401—416)

7. 0.05 (Frames 417—426)

8. xxiiss (Frames 455—459)

9. x (Frames 455—459)

10. 6 (Frames 455—459)

APPLICATIONS TO SOLUTIONS AND DOSES

Where modern facilities are available, the pharmacist often prepares medication for the patient in exactly the form in which it is to be administered. The nurse never assumes the responsibilities of the pharmacist. Why, then, does the nurse need to be able to solve problems in dosages and solutions? There are many reasons. Even in the modern hospital, nurses may carry out mathematical calculations to prepare doses or solutions according to doctors' orders or to detect errors before any harm may be done. Computation is also important for accurate collection of data and record-keeping; an increased efficiency results from the ability to calculate correctly. Of course, the most modern facilities are not always available, and a nurse should be prepared to handle a variety of different situations with confidence.

After completion of this section the student should be able to:

1. Find the strength of a solution in ratio or percent form, given the amount of solution and the amount of pure drug in the solution.

2. Find the amount of pure drug in a specified amount of solution of given strength.

3. Find the amount of liquid to add to a given amount of liquid, powder or tablets to make a required solution.

4. Find the number of tablets needed to make a specified amount of solution from given tablets.

5. Find the amount of a given solution or quantity of tablets to use for a prescribed dose.

PROFICIENCY GAUGE

To measure your proficiency, work out the following exercises. Uncover the printed answers only after you have answered all the questions.

1. Find the ratio strength of a pint of boric acid solution containing 20 Gm. of boric acid.

2. Find the percent strength in Item 1, above.

3. Find the amount of glycerin in f $\bar{3}$ lx of a 25% solution of glycerin.

4. How much magnesium sulfate is necessary for a preparation of f $\bar{3}$ x of a 1:5 solution?

5. How many gr. x tablets of sodium bicarbonate will be needed to make 1 L. of a 1% solution?

6. From boric acid solution, 1:400, how can you prepare 40 ounces of boric acid solution, 1:500?

7. Methadone hydrochloride is available in vials of solution containing 10 mg. per ml. How much solution should be used for a dose of 7 mg?

8. You have on hand a solution containing 3,000,000 units of penicillin per 5.0 ml. How much would you give a patient whose doctor has ordered a dose of 300,000 units?

9. Suppose that 3 quarts of a 1:2000 solution of potassium permanganate were needed and 0.2 Gm. scored tablets were on hand. How many tablets should be used?

10. If a normal adult dose of drug K is 0.6 Gm., find the dose for a child who weighs 60 pounds.

. . . .

Answers

1. 1:25

2. 4%

3. f ℥ xvi

4. ℥ ii

5. 15 tablets

6. Combine 32 ounces of boric acid solution, 1:400, with 8 ounces of water.

7. 0.7 ml.

8. 0.5 ml.

9. $7\frac{1}{2}$

10. 240 mg.

Read page 3 for instructions if you have not already done so.

Strength of a Solution

The ratio of amount of pure drug in a solution to the total amount of the solution is called the strength of the solution. It may be given in fraction form or percent form.

460. If 1 ounce of boric acid powder is dissolved in 499 ounces of water, how many ounces of solution are there altogether? What is the ratio of ounces of boric acid to ounces of solution? This ratio is called the strength of the boric acid solution.

. . . .

500; $\frac{1}{500}$ or 1:500

One ounce of boric acid added to 499 ounces of water yields 500 ounces of solution.

$$\frac{ounces\ of\ boric\ acid}{ounces\ of\ solution} = \frac{1}{500}$$

460a.

If you combine 25 ounces of glycerin with 75 ounces of water, how many ounces of solution do you have? What is the ratio of ounces of glycerin to ounces of solution; i.e., what is the strength of the solution?

. . . .

100; $\frac{1}{4}$ or 1:4

25 + 75 = 100 ounces of solution

$$\frac{ounces\ of\ glycerin}{ounces\ of\ solution} = \frac{25}{100} = \frac{1}{4}$$

461. Find the strength of the boric acid solution given in Frame 460 in percent form.

. . . .

0.2%

$$\frac{1}{500} = x\%, \quad \frac{1}{500} = \frac{x}{100}, \quad x = 0.2$$

462. Find the strength of the glycerin solution given in Frame 460a in percent form.

. . . .

25%

$$\frac{25}{100} = 25\%$$

463. A solution for injection of streptomycin sulfate contains 1 Gm. of drug in 2 ml. of solution. Find the strength of the solution in percent form.

. . . .

50%   *1 Gm. of drug is approximately equivalent to 1 ml.*

$$\frac{amount\ of\ drug\ in\ ml.}{amount\ of\ solution\ in\ ml.} = \frac{1.}{2} = 50\%$$

464. Each 1.5 ml. of an oleandomycin solution contained 100 mg. of the antibiotic. In ratio form, what was the strength of the solution?

. . . .

$\frac{1}{15}$ $\frac{amount\ of\ drug\ in\ ml.}{amount\ of\ solution\ in\ ml.} = \frac{0.1}{1.5} = \frac{1}{15}$

465. If you have 500 ounces of boric acid solution, 1:500, how much boric acid powder and how much water are present in the solution?

. . . .

1 ounce, 499 ounces

465a.

If you have 100 ounces of a $\frac{25}{100}$ solution of glycerin, how much glycerin and how much water are present?

. . . .

25 ounces glycerin and 75 ounces water

466. If you have 50 ounces of boric acid solution, 1 : 500, the quantity of boric acid powder present must be (less than/equal to/greater than) 1 ounce.

. . . .

less than

In Frame 465, we observed that in 500 ounces of solution, there was 1 ounce of powder present. In only 50 ounces of solution, then, there could not be as much as 1 ounce of powder.

---

467. If you have 400 ounces of boric acid solution, 1:200, the quantity of boric acid powder present must be (less than/equal to/greater than) 1 ounce.

. . . .

greater than

In a 1:200 solution, there is one ounce of powder in 200 ounces of solution. In 400 ounces of solution, there must be more than 1 ounce of powder.

---

468. If you have 120 ounces of a $^{25}/_{100}$ solution of glycerin, the amount of glycerin present in the solution must be (less than/equal to/greater than) 25 ounces.

. . . .

greater than

In 100 ounces of solution, there are 25 ounces of glycerin. In 120 ounces there must be more than 25 ounces of glycerin.

---

469. If you have 8 ounces of an alcohol solution, 7:10, the amount of alcohol present in the solution must be (less than/equal to/greater than) 7 ounces.

. . . .

less than

In 10 ounces of solution, there would be 7 ounces of alcohol. In only 8 ounces of solution, there must be less than 7 ounces of alcohol.

---

470. Given boric acid solution, 1:500, how many ounces of boric acid are present in 40 ounces of solution? Hint: Set up a table that can be converted to a proportion.

ounces of boric acid	x	1
ounces of solution	40	500

thus $\dfrac{\text{ounces of boric acid}}{\text{ounces of solution}} = \dfrac{x}{40} = \dfrac{1}{500}$.

Now solve the proportion.

. . . .

$\dfrac{2}{25}$

$$\dfrac{x}{40} = \dfrac{1}{500}$$

$$\dfrac{x}{40} \times 40 = \dfrac{1}{500} \times 40$$

$$x = \dfrac{4}{50} = \dfrac{2}{25}$$

---

471. How much boric acid is present in 75 ounces of boric acid solution, 1:500? Set up a table, write a proportion, and solve.

. . . .

$\dfrac{3}{20}$ ounce

$$\dfrac{ounces\ of\ boric\ acid}{ounces\ of\ solution} = \dfrac{x}{75} = \dfrac{1}{500}$$

$$x = \dfrac{1}{500} \times 75$$

$$x = \dfrac{3}{20}$$

---

472. How many ounces of glycerin are present in 8 ounces of a 25% solution of glycerin?

. . . .

2 ounces

---

473. An alcohol solution was made of 7 parts alcohol to 3 parts water. Find the ratio of alcohol to solution. How many ounces of alcohol were there in 50 ounces of solution?

. . . .

35 ounces

$$\dfrac{7}{7 + 3} = \dfrac{7}{10} = 7:10$$

$$\dfrac{7}{10} \times 50 = 35$$

---

474. A certain solution was made up of 2 parts drug to 3 parts water. How many ounces of drug are there in 60 ounces of solution?

. . . .

24 ounces

$$\dfrac{2}{5} \times 60 = 24$$

---

475. How many ounces of sodium biphosphate are present in 4 ounces of a 16% solution of sodium biphosphate?

. . . .

0.64 ounces

476. The doctor prescribes 25 ounces of saturated boric acid solution. This means a 55:1000 solution. In the 25 ounces, how much boric acid should be used?

. . . .

1⅜

$$\frac{ounces\ of\ boric\ acid}{ounces\ of\ solution} = \frac{x}{25} = \frac{55}{1000}$$

$$x = \frac{55}{1000} \times 25 = \frac{55}{40}\ or\ 1\tfrac{3}{8}$$

477. How much magnesium sulfate is necessary for a preparation of 10 ounces of a 1:2 solution?

. . . .

5 ounces

$$\frac{ounces\ of\ magnesium\ sulfate}{ounces\ of\ solution} = \frac{x}{10} = \frac{1}{2}$$

$$x = \frac{1}{2} \times 10;\ \ x = 5$$

478. How much full-strength cresol must be dissolved in water to prepare 5 ounces of saponated solution of cresol, 1:20?

. . . .

$\frac{1}{4}$ ounce

$$\frac{ounces\ of\ cresol}{ounces\ of\ solution} = \frac{x}{5} = \frac{1}{20}$$

$$x = \frac{1}{20} \times 5$$

$$x = \frac{1}{4}$$

479. What steps should be followed to find the quantity of drug in a solution?

. . . .

Multiply the strength of the solution (in ratio or percent form) by the number of units of solution.

---

480. How many ounces of glycerin are there in 30 ounces of a 60% solution of glycerin?

. . . .

18

Replace 60% by $\dfrac{60}{100}$.

$$\frac{number\ of\ ounces\ of\ glycerin}{number\ of\ ounces\ of\ solution} = \frac{x}{30} = \frac{60}{100}$$

$$x = \frac{60}{100} \times 30$$

$$= \frac{6}{10} \times 30$$

$$= 6 \times 3 = 18$$

---

481. How many ounces of sodium biphosphate are present in 8 ounces of a 20% solution of sodium biphosphate?

. . . .

$1\frac{3}{5}$

$$\frac{number\ of\ ounces\ of\ sodium\ biphosphate}{number\ of\ ounces\ of\ solution} =$$

$$\frac{x}{8} = \frac{20}{100}$$

$$x = \frac{20}{100} \times 8$$

$$= \frac{1}{5} \times 8$$

$$= \frac{8}{5}\ or\ 1\frac{3}{5}$$

Preparation of Solutions

Sometimes it is necessary to prepare solutions from given liquids, powder, or tablets. The given liquid may already be a solution to be diluted or it may be a pure drug. Labels or package inserts give specific details and instructions.

482. Suppose a dilute solution must be prepared from a stock solution. You may have on hand boric acid, 1:400, but a patient requires 20 ounces of boric acid, 1:500. What procedure would you follow? Hint: In this case, 2 tables that can be converted to 2 proportions would be helpful. Determine the number of ounces (x) of boric acid in 20 ounces of the desired solution, 1 : 500. Then find out how many ounces (y) of stock solution, 1:400 must be used.

. . . .

To 16 ounces of stock solution, add 4 ounces of water to get 20 ounces of solution.

Table I

ounces of boric acid	x	1
ounces of desired solution	20	500

Proportion I: $\dfrac{x}{20} = \dfrac{1}{500}$

Multiply both sides by 20:

$$x = \frac{1}{500} \times 20 = \frac{1}{25} = 0.04$$

Thus 0.04 ounce of boric acid will be present in the desired solution.

Table II

ounces of boric acid	0.04	1
ounces of stock solution needed	y	400

Proportion II: $\dfrac{0.04}{y} = \dfrac{1}{400}$

set product of means = product of extremes:

$$y = 0.04 \times 400 = 16$$

483. You may have on hand boric acid, 1:400, but a patient requires 50 ounces of boric acid, 1:500. What procedure would you follow? Hint: Determine the number of ounces (x) of boric acid in 50 ounces of the desired solution, 1:500. Then find out how many ounces (y) of stock solution, 1:400 must be used.

. . . .

Add 10 ounces of water to 40 ounces of boric acid to reach the 50 ounces desired.

Table I

ounces of boric acid	x	1
ounces of solution desired	50	500

Proportion I: $\dfrac{x}{50} = \dfrac{1}{500}$

Multiply both sides by 50:

$$x = \frac{1}{500} \times 50 = \frac{1}{10} = 0.1$$

Thus $\frac{1}{10}$ ounce of boric acid will be present in the desired solution.

Table II

ounces of boric acid	0.1	1
ounces of stock solution needed	y	400

Proportion II: $\dfrac{0.1}{y} = \dfrac{1}{400}$

Solve by multiplying means and extremes:

$y = 0.1 \times 400 = 40$

483a.

Check the results of Frame 483. Will 40 ounces of stock solution, 1:400, have the same amount of boric acid as 50 ounces of diluted solution, 1:500?

. . . .

Yes, since $\dfrac{1}{400} \times 40 = 0.01 = \dfrac{1}{500} \times 50$.

484. If you have a 55:1000 stock solution of boric acid and you need 25 ounces of a 1:500 solution, what procedure would you follow?

. . . .

Add enough water to the 1 ounce (rounded from $^{10}/_{11}$ ounce) of stock solution until 25 ounces is reached.

First step: How many ounces (x) of boric acid are present in 25 ounces of a 1:500 solution?

$$\frac{number\ of\ ounces\ of\ boric\ acid}{number\ of\ ounces\ of\ desired\ solution} =$$

$$\frac{x}{25} = \frac{1}{500}$$

$x = \dfrac{1}{500} \times 25 = \dfrac{1}{20}$ *ounce present in desired solution.*

Second step: How many ounces (y) of stock solution (55:1000) must be used?

$$\frac{number\ of\ ounces\ of\ boric\ acid}{number\ of\ ounces\ of\ stock\ solution} =$$

$$\frac{^1/_{20}}{y} = \frac{55}{1000}$$

Solve by multiplying means and extremes:

$$55y = \frac{1}{\cancel{20}_1} \times \cancel{1000}^{50}$$

$$y = \frac{50}{55} = \frac{10}{11} \ ounce$$

484a.

Check the results of Frame 484. Will 1 ounce of stock solution, $\dfrac{55}{1000}$, have about the same amount of boric acid as 25 ounces of diluted solution, 1:500?

. . . .

Yes, since $\dfrac{1}{500} \times 25 = \dfrac{25}{500} = \dfrac{50}{1000}$.

485. If you have a 55:1000 stock solution of boric acid and you need 10 ounces of a 1:500 solution, what procedure would you follow?

. . . .

$\frac{1}{2}$ ounce (rounded from $^4/_{11}$ ounce) of stock solution should be combined with enough water to make 10 ounces of desired solution.

$x =$ number of ounces of boric acid present in desired solution.

$$\frac{x}{10} = \frac{1}{500}$$

$x = \frac{1}{500} \times 10 = \frac{1}{50}$ ounce of boric acid needed.

$y =$ number of ounces of stock solution needed.

$$\frac{^1/_{50}}{y} = \frac{55}{1000}$$

$$55y = \frac{1}{\cancel{50}_1} \times \cancel{1000}^{20}$$

$y = \frac{20}{55} = \frac{4}{11}$ ounce of stock solution needed.

486. Intranasal solutions of phenylephrine, 1:400, may be administered to infants with colds so that they can breathe freely while nursing. An 8-ounce container of phenylephrine, 1:400, is to be prepared for the pediatric ward from the stock solution, 1:100, which is used for adults. How would you proceed?

. . . .

To 2 ounces of stock solution add enough water to make 8 ounces of desired solution.

Let $x =$ number of ounces of phenylephrine in the required 8 ounces of solution.

$$\frac{x}{8} = \frac{1}{400}; \quad x = \frac{1}{400} \times 8$$

$x = \frac{1}{50}$ ounce of phenylephrine needed.

Let $y =$ number of ounces of stock solution that should be used.

$$\frac{^1/_{50}}{y} = \frac{1}{100}$$

$$100 \times \frac{1}{50} = y$$

$y = 2$, since the product of the means = the product of the extremes.

487. To prepare an enema, $4\frac{1}{2}$ fluid ounces of sodium phosphate, 6:100, are needed. On hand is sodium phosphate, 2:15. How would you proceed?

. . . .

To 2 ounces (rounded from 2.025 ounces) of stock solution, add enough water to make a total of $4\frac{1}{2}$ fluid ounces.

Let x = number of ounces of sodium phosphate in the required $4\frac{1}{2}$ ounces of solution.

$$\frac{x}{4\frac{1}{2}} = \frac{6}{100}$$

$$x = \frac{6}{100} \times 4\frac{1}{2}$$

$$x = \frac{6}{100} \times \frac{9}{2} = 0.06 \times 4.5$$

$x = 0.27$ ounce of sodium phosphate needed.

Let y = number of ounces of stock solution that should be used.

$$\frac{0.27}{y} = \frac{2}{15}$$

$$2y = 0.27 \times 15 = 4.05$$

$$y = 2.025$$

488. From a 6% stock solution of sodium phosphate, how can you prepare 8 ounces of a 5% sodium phosphate solution? Hint: Use 2 proportions, one for the desired solution and one for the stock solution, as in Frames 482 through 487.

. . . .

Add water to 7 ounces (rounded from $6\frac{2}{3}$ ounces) of solution until you have 8 ounces.

Let x = number of ounces of sodium phosphate required in the desired solution.

$$\frac{x}{8} = \frac{5}{100}; \ x = 0.05 \times 8 = 0.4$$

Let y = number of ounces of stock solution to be used.

$$\frac{0.4}{y} = 0.06$$

product of means = product of extremes

$$6y = 0.4 \times 100; \ 6y = 40; \ y = \frac{40}{6}, \frac{20}{3}, \text{ or } 6\frac{2}{3}$$

489. How much of a 25% solution would be needed to prepare 10 ounces of a 20% solution?

. . . .

8 ounces

Let x = number of ounces of drug needed in the 20% solution.

$$\frac{x}{10} = \frac{20}{100}$$

$x = 2$

Let y = number of ounces of drug in the 25% solution.

$$\frac{2}{y} = \frac{25}{100} = \frac{1}{4}$$

Since the product of the means = product of the extremes, $y = 8$.

490. How much of a 20% stock solution would be needed to prepare 80 fluid ounces of a 1:25 solution?

. . . .

16 ounces

Let x = number of ounces of drug in desired solution.

$$\frac{x}{80} = \frac{1}{25}$$

$$x = \frac{1}{25} \times 80 = 0.04 \times 80$$

$x = 3.2$ ounces of drug required in the 1:25 solution.

Let y = number of ounces of stock solution to be used.

$$\frac{3.2}{y} = \frac{20}{100}, \text{ but } \frac{20}{100} = \frac{1}{5}, \text{ so that}$$

$$\frac{3.2}{y} = \frac{1}{5}$$

$y = 3.2 \times 5$

$y = 16$ ounces of the 20% solution

491. How much of a 15% solution should be used to prepare 6 ounces of a 2:3 solution?

. . . .

$26\frac{2}{3}$

Let x = number of ounces of drug in desired solution.

$$\frac{x}{6} = \frac{2}{3}$$

$$x = \frac{2}{3} \times 6$$

x = 4 ounces of drug needed in the desired solution.

Let y = number of ounces of stock solution to be used.

$\frac{4}{y} = \frac{15}{100}$, but $\frac{15}{100} = \frac{3}{20}$ so that $\frac{4}{y} = \frac{3}{20}$

$3y = 80$ and $y = \frac{80}{3}$ or $26\frac{2}{3}$ ounces

492. How many 2 mg. tablets of reserpine will be needed to make 4 cc. of 1:400 solution?

. . . .

5 tablets

Let x = number of cc. of drug in desired solution.

$$\frac{\text{cc. of drug}}{\text{cc. of solution}} = \frac{x}{4} = \frac{1}{400}$$

$x = \frac{1}{400} \times 4 = 0.01$ cc. or 0.01 ml.

Now 0.01 ml. weighs about 0.01 Gm. Change 0.01 Gm. to 10 mg. If each tablet contains 2 mg., the number of tablets needed is $\frac{10}{2} = 5$.

493. How would you prepare 0.2 ml. of a 10% solution of prednisolone acetate using 5 mg. tablets?

. . . .

dissolve 4 tablets

Let x = number of ml. of drug in desired solution.

$$\frac{ml.\ of\ drug}{ml.\ of\ solution} = \frac{x}{0.2} = 0.10$$

$x = 0.2 \times 0.10 = 0.02$

Thus 0.02 ml. of drug is needed or 0.02 Gm. or 20 mg. If each tablet contains 5 mg., the number of tablets needed is 4.

---

494. If 1 quart of 1:2000 solution of potassium permanganate were needed to wash out a stomach and 0.2 Gm. scored tablets were on hand, how would you proceed?

. . . .

dissolve $2\frac{1}{2}$ tablets
using enough water
to reach 1 quart

Let x = number of Gm. of drug in desired solution. Replace 1 quart by 1000 Gm.

$$\frac{Gm.\ of\ drug}{Gm.\ of\ solution} = \frac{x}{1000} = \frac{1}{2000}, \ x = \frac{1}{2} = 0.5$$

Thus 0.5 Gm. of drug is needed. If each tablet has 0.2 Gm., the number of tablets needed is $\frac{0.5}{0.2} = \frac{5}{2} = 2\frac{1}{2}$.

---

495. In how much water should a 2-Gm. tablet of drug *P* be dissolved in order to have a 1:4 solution?

. . . .

6 ml.

Let x = number of ml. of solution. A 2-Gm. tablet will provide about 2 ml. of solution.

$$\frac{ml.\ of\ drug}{ml.\ of\ solution} = \frac{2}{x} = \frac{1}{4}$$

$x = 2 \times 4 = 8$

A total of 8 ml. of solution is needed, of which 2 ml. will be pure drug. Thus 6 ml. of water should be used.

496. Answer the same question for a 10% solution.

· · · · · · · · · · · ·

18 ml.

$$\frac{2}{x} = \frac{1}{10}, \quad x = 20$$

A total of 20 ml. of solution is needed, of which 2 ml. will be pure drug. Thus 18 ml. of water should be used.

497. In how much water should a 0.3 Gm. tablet of drug Q be dissolved in order to have a 0.8% solution?

· · · · · · · · · · · ·

37.2 ml.

Let x = number of ml. of solution. A 3-Gm. tablet will provide about 3 ml. of solution.

$$\frac{ml.\ of\ drug}{ml.\ of\ solution} = \frac{.3}{x} = \frac{.8}{100} = \frac{8}{1000}$$

8x = 300, x = 37.5

Of a total of 37.5 ml. of solution, 0.3 ml. will be the volume of the drug. Thus 37.2 ml. of water are needed.

498. In each of the following cases, water is to be added to the given amount of drug to make the specified solution. Fill in the blanks in the chart.

	Amount of Drug	Strength of Solution Required	Amount of Water to Be Added
(a)	pt. i	1:4	
(b)	1 Gm. tablet	0.1%	
(c)	10 ml.		20 ml.
(d)	f ℥ ii	50%	
(e)	gr. $\frac{1}{4}$	1:25	
(f)	5 ml.		15 ml.
(g)	℥ iii	1:5	

· · · · · · · · · · · ·

(a)	pt. i	1 : 4	pt. iii
(b)	1 Gm. tablet	0.1%	999 ml.
(c)	10 ml.	1 : 3 = 33%	20 ml.
(d)	f ℥ ii	50%	f ℥ ii
(e)	gr. $\frac{1}{4}$	1 : 25	ℳ vi
(f)	5 ml.	1 : 4 = 25%	15 ml.
(g)	℥ iii	1 : 5	℥ xii

In each case, let

$$\frac{amount\ of\ drug}{amount\ of\ solution} = strength\ of\ solution$$

(a) $\frac{1}{x} = \frac{1}{4}, \quad x = 4$

To make 4 pints of solution with 1 pint of drug, use 3 pints of water.

(b) $\frac{1}{x} = \frac{0.1}{100} = \frac{1}{1000}, \quad x = 1000$

To make 1000 ml. = 1 L. of solution, with a 1-Gm. tablet, use 999 ml. of water.

(c) $\frac{10}{10 + 20} = \frac{10}{30} = 1 : 3\ or\ 33\%$

(d) $\frac{2}{x} = \frac{1}{2}, \quad x = 4$

(e) $\frac{1/4}{x} = \frac{1}{25}, \quad x = \frac{25}{4} = 6\frac{1}{4}$

(f) $\frac{5}{5 + 15} = \frac{5}{20} = 1 : 4\ or\ 25\%$

(g) $\frac{3}{x} = \frac{1}{5}, \quad x = 15$

Preparation of Doses Using Solutions

499. To carry out a doctor's orders for a prescribed dose, a nurse may have to calculate the amount of solution to administer from stock on hand. The same principle is used throughout:

$$\frac{quantity\ of\ solution\ needed}{quantity\ of\ solution\ available} = \frac{quantity\ of\ pure\ drug\ needed}{quantity\ of\ pure\ drug\ in\ available\ solution}$$

Each 2.0 ml. vial of benzathine penicillin G contains 1,200,000 units. How many ml. should be given to a patient needing 600,000 units?

. . . .

1.0 ml.

$$\frac{ml.\ of\ solution\ needed}{ml.\ of\ solution\ in\ vial} = \frac{units\ of\ drug\ needed}{units\ of\ drug\ in\ vial}$$

$$\frac{x}{2.0} = \frac{600,000}{1,200,000}$$

$$\frac{x}{2.0} = \frac{1}{2}, \quad x = 1.0$$

500. Streptomycin sulfate injection is packed in a 2.5-cc. vial, equivalent to 1.0 Gm. streptomycin base. An elderly patient is to be given 0.4 Gm. What part of the vial should be used?

. . . .

1.0 cc.

$$\frac{cc.\ of\ solution\ needed}{cc.\ of\ solution\ in\ vial} = \frac{Gm.\ of\ drug\ needed}{Gm.\ of\ drug\ in\ vial}$$

$$\frac{x}{2.5} = \frac{0.4}{1}$$

$$x = 1.0$$

---

501. Terramycin intramuscular solution is available in 2 cc. prescored glass ampules containing 250 mg./2 cc. A doctor's orders for a young patient call for doses of 60 mg. every 8 hours. What part of the ampule would be used for each dose?

. . . .

0.5 cc.

$$\frac{cc.\ needed}{cc.\ in\ ampule} = \frac{mg.\ needed}{mg.\ in\ ampule}$$

$$\frac{x}{2} = \frac{6\emptyset}{25\emptyset}$$

$$x = \frac{12}{25} = \frac{1}{2} = 0.5\ (rounded\ from\ \frac{12}{25})$$

---

502. Use of intramuscular bacitracin is limited to the treatment of infants with pneumonia caused by staphylococci shown to be susceptible to the drug. It is supplied in 50 cc. of solution containing 50,000 units. The doctor ordered a dose of 400 units/kg. for a 10-pound infant. How many units would you give? How many cc. of solution would you give?

. . . .

1800 units; 1.8 cc.

$$\frac{x\ (child's\ weight\ in\ kg.)}{1\ kg.} = \frac{10\ lb.}{2.2\ lbs.};$$

$$x = 4.5\ in\ kg.$$

$$Dose = 400 \times 4.5 = 1800\ units$$

$$\frac{x\ (cc.\ needed)}{50\ (cc.\ available)} =$$

$$\frac{18\emptyset\emptyset\ (units\ needed)}{50,0\emptyset\emptyset\ (units\ in\ available\ solution)}$$

$$x = 1.8\ in\ cc.$$

503. Fill in the blanks. Assume that orders have been given for specific drugs and that solutions containing those drugs are on hand as indicated.

Doctors' Orders	Label on Container of Solution	Amount of Solution to Be Administered
6,000 units	20,000 units/ml.	(a)
gr. $\frac{1}{12}$	ℳ xx = gr. $\frac{1}{4}$	(b)
80 mg.	50 mg. in 2.0 cc.	(c)
200,000 units	1,000,000 units/10.0 ml.	(d)
0.04 gram	0.5 gram in 1.8 cc.	(e)

. . . .

(a) 0.3 ml.

(a) $\dfrac{x \ (ml. \ needed)}{1 \ (ml. \ on \ hand)} = \dfrac{6,000 \ (units \ needed)}{20,000 \ (units \ on \ hand)}$

$x = 0.3$

(b) ℳ vii

(b) $\dfrac{x \ (minims \ needed)}{20 \ (minims)} = \dfrac{^1/_{12} \ (grain \ needed)}{^1/_4 \ (grain)}$

$\dfrac{x}{20} = \dfrac{1}{12} \times 4 = \dfrac{1}{3}$

$x = \dfrac{20}{3} = 6\dfrac{2}{3}$

(c) 3.2 cc.

(c) $\dfrac{x \ (cc. \ needed)}{2.0 \ (cc.)} = \dfrac{80 \ (mg. \ needed)}{50 \ (mg.)}$

$x = \dfrac{16}{5} = 3\dfrac{1}{5}$

(d) 2 ml.

(d) $\dfrac{x \ (ml. \ needed)}{10 \ (ml. \ on \ hand)} =$

$\dfrac{200,000 \ (units \ needed)}{1,000,000 \ (units \ on \ hand)}$

$x = \dfrac{20}{10} = 2$

(e) 0.1 cc.

(e) $\dfrac{x \ (cc. \ needed)}{1.8 \ (cc. \ on \ hand)} = \dfrac{0.04 \ (Gm. \ needed)}{0.5 \ (Gm. \ on \ hand)}$

$x = \dfrac{(0.4 \times (1.8)}{5} = \dfrac{0.72}{5} = 0.144$

Preparation of Doses Using Tablets

504. A dose in the form of a solution is to be prepared containing gr. $\frac{1}{100}$ of a drug. On hand are tablets gr. $\frac{1}{200}$. How many tablets should be used?

. . . .

2

$$\frac{x \text{ (tablets needed)}}{1 \text{ (tablet of known strength)}} =$$

$$\frac{1/100 \text{ (grains needed)}}{1/200 \text{ (grains in 1 tablet)}} = \frac{1}{100} \times 200 = 2$$

505. Solve the same problem if tablets gr. $\frac{1}{150}$ are on hand.

. . . .

$1\frac{1}{2}$

$$\frac{x}{1} = \frac{1/100}{1/150} = \frac{1}{100} \times 150 = \frac{15}{10} = 1\frac{1}{2}$$

506. How many tablets of 0.02 Gm. are needed for a dose of gr. $\frac{1}{4}$?

. . . .

$\frac{3}{4}$ tablet

$$gr. \frac{1}{4} = 0.015 \text{ Gm. approximately}$$

$$\frac{x}{1} = \frac{0.015}{0.02} = \frac{15}{20} = \frac{3}{4}$$

507. According to the label, each tablet in the bottle weighs gr. $\frac{3}{4}$. The patient is required to have gr. $\frac{1}{2}$. What is the ratio of the required dose to the dose provided by a single tablet; that is, what part of the tablet should the patient have?

. . . .

$\frac{2}{3}$

$$\frac{1}{2} : \frac{3}{4} = \frac{1}{2} \div \frac{3}{4} = \frac{1}{2} \times \frac{4}{3} = \frac{2}{3}$$

508. Fill in the following table:

Dose Required	Label on Container of Tablets	Number of Tablets Needed
gr iii	gr iss	(a)
gr $\frac{1}{3}$	gr $\frac{1}{9}$	(b)
0.5 Gm.	0.2 Gm.	(c)
2.5 Gm.	1.2 Gm.	(d)
gr. iii	gr. xii	(e)
gr. xiv	0.5 Gm.	(f)
0.03 Gm.	gr. $\frac{1}{6}$	(g)

. . . .

(a) 2

(b) 3

(c) $2\frac{1}{2}$

(d) 2

(e) $\frac{1}{4}$

(f) 2

(g) 3

(a) $\frac{x}{1} = \frac{3}{1\frac{1}{2}} = 3 \times \frac{2}{3} = 2$

(b) $\frac{x}{1} = \frac{\frac{1}{3}}{\frac{1}{9}} = \frac{1}{3} \times 9 = 3$

(c) $\frac{x}{1} = \frac{0.5}{0.2} = \frac{5}{2} = 2\frac{1}{2}$

(d) $\frac{x}{1} = \frac{2.5}{1.2} = \frac{25}{12} = 2$

(e) $\frac{x}{1} = \frac{3}{12} = \frac{1}{4}$

(f) $\frac{x}{1} = \frac{14}{7\frac{1}{2}} = 14 \times \frac{2}{15} = 2$

(g) $\frac{x}{1} = \frac{0.03}{0.01} = 3$

Calculation of Doses for Children

509. In determining a dose for a child between 1 and 12 years of age, it is useful to know Young's rule:

Child's dose = $\dfrac{\text{child's age in years } (y)}{y + 12}$ × adult dose

This rule first requires us to find the ratio of the child's age in years to the age of an adult who is 12 years older than the child. Suppose Young's rule were to be used for an 8-year-old. Find the ratio of the child's age to the age of the adult who is 12 years older.

. . . .

2:5 $\dfrac{8}{20} = \dfrac{2}{5}$ or 2:5

---

510. Suppose Young's rule were to be used for a 10-year-old. Find the ratio of the child's age to the age of the adult who is 12 years older.

. . . .

5:11 $\dfrac{10}{22} = \dfrac{5}{11} =$ or 5:11

---

511. A child will usually receive a dose that is a proper fraction of the normal adult dose. If a normal adult dose is 0.1 Gm. of digitalis and a little girl is to receive $\dfrac{2}{5}$ of the adult dose, how much digitalis should she receive?

. . . .

40 mg. $\dfrac{\text{Fraction of}}{\text{adult dose}} = \dfrac{\text{child's}}{\text{dose}}$

                          $\dfrac{2}{5}$ × 0.1 Gm. = 0.04 Gm. or 40 mg.

---

512. Ferrous sulfate is to be given to a boy who should have $\dfrac{1}{3}$ of the adult dose of 0.9 Gm. per day. How many mg. should he receive per day?

. . . .

300 mg. $\dfrac{1}{3}$ × 0.9 = 0.3 Gm. or 300 mg.

513. The appropriate proper fractions to use in calculating a child's dose from an adult dose are found by the following rules:

Child's Age or Weight	Child's Dose (Fraction of Adult Dose)
0 – 11 months	$\dfrac{\text{Age in months}}{150} \times$ adult dose (Young's rule)
1 – 12 years	$\dfrac{\text{Age in years } (y)}{y + 12} \times$ adult dose (Fred's rule)
0 – 150 pounds	$\dfrac{\text{Weight in pounds}}{150} \times$ adult dose (Clark's rule)

What fraction of an adult dose should be given to a child who weighs 30 kg.?

. . . .

$\dfrac{11}{25}$

30 kg. = 66 lbs. approximately

$$\frac{66}{150} = \frac{11}{25}$$

514. Suppose the adult dose of a drug is 0.6 Gm. Find the doses to be given to the following children: Carl, who weighs 40 pounds; Yolanda, who is 3 months old; Fred, who is 9 years old.

. . . .

Carl: 160 mg.

$$\frac{40}{150} \times 0.6 = \frac{4 \times 0.6}{15} = \frac{4 \times 0.2}{5} = \frac{0.8}{5} =$$
$$0.16 \ or \ 160 \ mg.$$

Yolanda: 12 mg.

$$\frac{3}{150} \times 0.6 = \frac{0.6}{50} = 0.012 \ or \ 12 \ mg.$$

Fred: 260 mg.

$$\frac{9}{21} \times 0.6 = \frac{3}{7} \times 0.6 = \frac{1.8}{7} = 0.26$$

515. Find the doses in mg. for Carl, Yolanda, and Fred, assuming that the adult dose is gr. $\dfrac{1}{6}$.

. . . .

Replace gr. $\frac{1}{6}$ by 10 mg.

Carl: 2.7 mg.

$$\frac{40}{150} \times 10 = \frac{40}{15} = 2.7$$

Yolanda: 0.2 mg.

$$\frac{3}{150} \times 10 = \frac{3}{15} = 0.2$$

Fred: 4.3 mg.

$$\frac{9}{21} \times 10 = \frac{30}{7} = 4.3$$

Calculation of Doses Based on Body Weight

516. Medication is sometimes ordered in mg. per kg. of body weight. How much atropine would you give a child weighing 10 kg. if orders called for 0.01 mg. per kg.?

. . . .

0.1 mg.

$10 \times 0.01 = 0.1$

---

517. How much atropine would you give a child weighing 30 lbs. if orders were as in Frame 516?

. . . .

0.14 mg.

First, the child's weight in kg. must be calculated:

1 kg. = 2.2 (approximately)

x kg. = 30 lbs.

x:1 = 30:2.2

x = 30 ÷ 2.2 = 14

Then 0.01 × 14 = 0.14

---

518. For intramuscular administration, neomycin sulfate is ordered in doses of 10 — 15 mg. per kg. of body weight per day, not to exceed a total of 1 Gm. daily. If a patient weighs 220 pounds, how much neomycin sulfate should he receive per day?

. . . .

1 Gm.

2.2 lbs. = 1 kg.

220 lbs. = 100 kg.

10 mg. for each kg. requires 10 × 100
*   = 1000 mg. = 1 Gm.*

15 mg. for each kg. requires 15 × 100
*   = 1500 mg. = 1.5 Gm.*

SUMMARY

1. Ratio strength of a solution $= \dfrac{\text{amount of pure drug in the solution}}{\text{total amount of solution}}$, where measurements are made in the same units.
   Percent strength of a solution = ratio strength × 100%.

   Example: Boric acid solution made from 1 ounce of boric acid powder and 399 ounces of water has ratio strength $\dfrac{1}{400}$, also written as 1:400. The percent strength is $\dfrac{1}{4}$% or 0.25%.

2. *Preparation of solutions.* If a stock solution is to be diluted to a solution of desired strength, solve two proportions:

   First: $\dfrac{\text{amount } (x) \text{ of pure drug desired in solution}}{\text{total amount of desired solution}} = $ ratio strength of desired solution

   Second: $\dfrac{\text{amount of pure drug desired}}{\text{total amount } (y) \text{ of stock solution needed}} = $ ratio strength of stock solution

   Similar reasoning is used if tablets are to be dissolved to make a solution.

   Example: Boric acid, 1:400, is to be diluted in order to prepare 20 ounces of boric acid, 1:500.

   First: $\dfrac{x}{20} = \dfrac{1}{500}$, $x = 0.04$ (quantity of boric acid needed)

   Second: $\dfrac{0.04}{y} = \dfrac{1}{400}$, $y = 16$ (quantity of stock solution needed)

   Therefore combine 16 ounces of boric acid, 1:400, with 4 ounces of water to make 20 ounces of boric acid, 1:500.

   Example: Suppose 4 ml. of boric acid 1:400 were to be prepared with 0.002-Gm. tablets.

   First: $\dfrac{x}{4} = \dfrac{1}{400}$, $x = 0.01$ ml. (quantity of boric acid needed)

   Second: $\dfrac{0.01}{x} = \dfrac{0.002}{1}$, $x = \dfrac{0.01}{0.002} = 5$ (number of tablets needed)

   If 0.01 Gm. are subdivided into tablets of 0.002 Gm. each, 5 tablets are necessary.

3. *Preparation of doses.* To calculate how much solution to measure for a prescribed dose from a given amount of solution on hand, solve the proportion:

   $\dfrac{\text{quantity of solution needed}}{\text{quantity of solution on hand}} = \dfrac{\text{quantity of pure drug needed}}{\text{quantity of pure drug in solution on hand}}$

Example: To calculate how much solution to measure for a dose of 0.4 Gm. from a 2.5-cc. vial containing 1.0 Gm. of drug, solve:

$$\frac{x}{2.5} = \frac{0.4}{1}, \quad x = 1.0$$

Therefore 1 cc. of solution should be measured.

To calculate a child's dose from an adult dose, multiply the appropriate fraction by the adult dose. Appropriate fractions: for an infant under 1 year, $\dfrac{\text{age in months}}{150}$; for a child from 1 to 12 years, $\dfrac{\text{age in years } (y)}{y + 12}$; and for a child who weighs less than 150 lbs., $\dfrac{\text{weight in lbs.}}{150}$.

Example: Assume the adult dose of a drug is 300 mg. Then

a baby of 4 months would receive $\dfrac{4}{150}$ X 300 mg. = 8 mg.;

a child of 3 years would receive $\dfrac{3}{15}$ X 300 mg. = 60 mg.; and

a child who weighs 50 lbs. would receive $\dfrac{50}{150}$ X 300 mg. = 100 mg.

Exercises for Extra Practice

Fill in the following tables:

1.

	Amount of Pure Drug	Amount of Water	Total Amount of Solution	Ratio Strength	Percentage Strength
(a)	℥ v		℥ xv		
(b)	100 mg.	49.9 ml.			
(c)	1 Gm.				50%
(d)			1.5 ml.	$\frac{1}{15}$	
(e)	gr. xxv			$\frac{1}{4}$	
(f)			40 ounces	1:200	
(g)		2.4 ml.	2.5 ml.		
(h)		30 ml.			5.5%
(i)		8 ml.			$\frac{1}{4}$%

2.

	Amount of Pure Drug	Strength of Solution	Total Amount of Solution	Strength of Tablets	Number of Tablets
(a)		1:500	4 cc.	2 mg.	
(b)		1%	0.4 ml.	2 mg.	
(c)			20 ml.	0.1 Gm.	4
(d)	2 mg.	$\frac{1}{300}$		0.3 mg.	
(e)	gr. $\frac{1}{2}$		1 ml.	gr. $\frac{1}{6}$	
(f)	gr. xxx	50%			2
(g)	0.6 Gm.		0.5 L.	gr. iv	

3. Calculate the child's dose in each of the following situations:

	Information About the Child	Usual Adult Dose
(a)	8 years	200 mg.
(b)	5 years	0.3 ml.
(c)	65 lbs.	10.5 units
(d)	4 months	gr. $\frac{1}{40}$
(e)	7 years	15 ml.
(f)	3 months	12 ounces
(g)	130 lbs.	18.3 mg.
(h)	80 lbs.	25,000 units

. . . .

Answers

	Amount of Pure Drug	Amount of Water	Total Amount of Solution	Ratio Strength	Percentage Strength
1. (a)	℥ v	f ℥ x	℥ xv	$\frac{1}{3}$	33%
(b)	100 mg.	49.9 ml.	50 ml.	$1:500 = \frac{1}{500}$	$\frac{1}{5}\% = 0.2\%$
(c)	1 Gm.	1 ml.	2 ml.	$\frac{1}{2}$	50%
(d)	0.1 Gm.	1.4 ml.	1.5 ml.	$\frac{1}{15}$	$\frac{100}{15}\% = 6\frac{2}{3}\%$
(e)	gr. xxv	4.5 ml.	6 ml.	$\frac{1}{4}$	25%
(f)	0.2 ounce	39.8 ounces	40 ounces	1:200	$\frac{1}{2}\%$
(g)	0.1 Gm.	2.4 ml.	2.5 ml.	1:25	4%

1. (h) 1.7 Gm.   30 ml.   31.7 ml.   55:1000   5.5%

   (i) 0.02 Gm.   8 ml.   8.02 ml.   1:400 $\frac{1}{4}$%

2. (a) Pure drug $= \frac{1}{500} \times 4 = 0.008$ ml. or 8 mg.; 4 tablets

   (b) Pure drug $= 4$ mg.; 2 tablets

   (c) Pure drug $= 0.4$ Gm.; strength $= 2\%$

   (d) Number of tablets $= \frac{2}{0.3} = 7$; amount of solution $= 0.6$ ml.

   (e) Number of tablets $= 3$; strength of solution $= \frac{\frac{1}{2}}{15} = \frac{1}{30}$

   (f) Amount of solution $= 4$ ml.; strength of tablets $=$ gr. xv

   (g) Strength of solution $= \frac{6}{5000} = 0.12\%$; $2\frac{1}{2}$ tablets

3. (a) $\frac{8}{20} \times 200$ mg. $= 80$ mg.   (b) $\frac{5}{17} \times 0.3$ ml. $= 0.1$ ml.

   (c) $\frac{65}{150} \times 10.5$ units $= 4.5$ units   (d) $\frac{4}{150} \times$ gr. $\frac{1}{40} =$ gr. $\frac{1}{1500}$ or 0.04 mg.

   (e) $\frac{7}{19} \times 15$ ml. $= 5.5$ ml.   (f) $\frac{3}{150} \times 12$ ounces $= 0.2$ ounce or 7 ml.

   (g) $\frac{130}{150} \times 18.3$ mg. $= 15.9$ mg.   (h) $\frac{80}{150} \times 25,000$ units $= 13,333$ units

INVENTORY

The set of exercises below will show you whether you are already an expert or whether you need a little more practice. If you do need more practice, the numbers next to the answers will direct you to the particular frames that should receive your special attention.

1. Find the ratio strength of 6 drams of silver nitrate solution containing 4 Gm. of silver nitrate.

2. Find the percent strength in Item 1, above.

3. Find the amount of reserpine in 2 ml. of a 1:400 solution.

4. How much drug is necessary for a preparation of f $\breve{5}$ xv of a 20% solution?

5. How many gr. $\dfrac{1}{5}$ tablets of reserpine will be needed to make 20 cc. of a 0.3% solution?

6. From boric acid solution, 1:300, how can you prepare 36 ounces of boric acid solution, 1:400?

7. Hydrocortisone acetate is available in a 5-cc. vial containing 50 mg. of drug per 2 cc. How many cc. should be used for a dose of 10 mg.?

8. From a solution containing 1,200,000 units of benzathine penicillin G per 2 ml., a dose of 900,000 units must be given. How many ml. should be used?

9. How many 5-mg. tablets would you dissolve in order to prepare 0.3 ml. of a 10% solution of drug Q?

10. Find the dose for a 4-month old baby if a normal adult dose of a certain drug is 0.6 Gm.

. . . .

Answers

1. $\dfrac{1}{6}$ or 1:6 (Frame 460)

2. $16\dfrac{2}{3}$% (Frame 461)

3. 5 mg. (Frame 465)

4. f $\breve{5}$ iii (Frame 472)

5. 5 tablets (Frames 492 and 508)

6. Use 27 ounces of boric acid solution 1:300 with 9 ounces of water to make 36 ounces of boric acid solution 1:400. (Frame 482)

7. 0.4 cc. (Frame 500)

8. 1.5 ml. (Frame 499)

9. 6 tablets (Frame 508)

10. 16 mg. (Frame 513)

THE POCKET CALCULATOR

A modern book on mathematical calculations would be incomplete without a section on the pocket calculator. It is a very handy device which can perform some of our work for us and help us check whatever calculations we do.

We cannot expect the calculator to do all of our work. It does not eliminate the need to understand the mathematical operations involved. The calculator carries out only the simplest operations and only after we decide what should be done and which keys to press. Thus, to solve our problems in drugs and solutions, we must decide what numbers and what operations to use and in what order. There are no keys on the calculator to tell us, say, which fraction is appropriate in a given situation, what fraction or mixed number is equivalent to a given fraction, or which of two fractions or decimals represents the larger quantity. It does not make use of tables of common equivalents.

What help can the calculator give us? If we enter numbers in decimal form, the machine can add, subtract, multiply, and divide them. Some models will also find percents. A calculator with a memory device will store results of our operations and retrieve them when we wish. Any of the models can be used to increase our speed in computation or simply to check results of our pencil and paper arithmetic. When several calculations are needed in the process of solving a problem, we have a choice of keeping intermediate results on paper or in the memory device of the calculator. Intermediate results may then be combined by paper and pencil or by the calculator to arrive at the final result. It is important to understand the mathematical techniques thoroughly in order to know what instructions to give the calculator and to check that our results make sense.

After completion of this section, the student should:

1. Be able to recognize the basic features of commonly used pocket calculators.

2. Be prepared with a list of questions to ask when shopping for a suitable model.

3. Be able to make appropriate use of the calculator in solving problems in nursing science.

Basic Features of a Pocket Calculator

519. Many different models are available, but those designed for general use have essentially the same features. The following diagram shows one possible arrangement of these features.

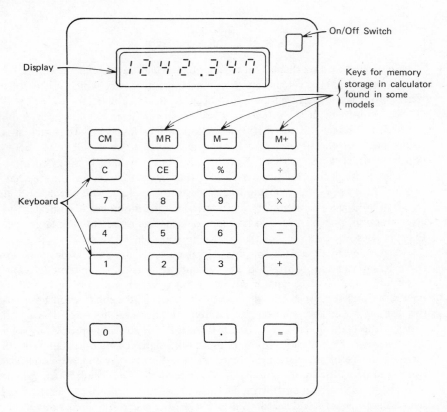

On the diagram above, find the keys to press for addition, subtraction, multiplication, and division.

520. By means of the keyboard, we can enter the numbers we need and the operations we mean to use, and we can clear the calculator for the next problem. By pointing to the diagram above, indicate steps in carrying out a problem such as 2 + 3 = ? Be sure to first use the clear key (c) to clear the machine of all previous calculations.

. . . .

c , 2 , + , 3 , = . The display will read 5 .

521. By pointing to the diagram to indicate which keys to press, try out a few simple exercises to get an idea of how a calculator is used. If you already own one, read carefully and use the instructions that accompany your calculator.

8.9 × 7.32 = _____

0.3 − 0.07 = _____

6 ÷ 5.3 = _____

700 ÷ 2.05 = _____

. . . .

[c] , [8] , [.] , [9] , [×] , [7] , [.] , [3] , [2] , [=] ; display will read [65.148]

[c] , [0] , [.] , [3] , [−] , [0] , [.] , [0] , [7] , [=] ; display will read [0.23]

[c] , [6] , [÷] , [5] , [.] , [3] , [=] ; display will read [1.1320754]

[c] , [7] , [0] , [0] , [÷] , [2] , [.] , [0] , [5] , [=] ; display will read [341.46341]

522. In the preceding illustrations, we have used the keys in the same order as the symbols appear in the equation. This is based on the assumption that the calculator uses "algebraic logic." Because some models follow other sequences, it is essential to study the manual of instructions accompanying the calculator. If $7 \times 3 \div 4 = x$, which of the following sequences for finding x is called algebraic logic?

(a) [c] , [7] , [3] , [×] , [4] , [÷] , [=]

(b) [c] , [7] , [×] , [3] , [÷] , [4] , [=]

. . . .

(b)

523. Find the memory keys ($\boxed{\text{CM}}$, $\boxed{\text{MR}}$, $\boxed{\text{M}-}$, $\boxed{\text{M}+}$) on the keyboard. They are useful in solving problems requiring two or more steps. To use a simple illustration, assume the solution of a problem requires the following steps:

(1) Find 2 + 3

(2) Find 4 + 5

(3) Multiply the results.

On a calculator, we might follow this sequence:

(1) $\boxed{\text{c}}$, $\boxed{\text{CM}}$, $\boxed{2}$, $\boxed{+}$, $\boxed{3}$, $\boxed{=}$, $\boxed{\text{M}+}$

(2) $\boxed{4}$, $\boxed{+}$, $\boxed{5}$, $\boxed{\times}$, $\boxed{\text{MR}}$, $\boxed{=}$

First, we clear the calculator, $\boxed{\text{c}}$, and the memory, $\boxed{\text{CM}}$; then we find 2 + 3 and store the result, $\boxed{\text{M}+}$. Second, we find 4 + 5, indicate the intent to multiply, $\boxed{\times}$, recall the first number $\boxed{\text{MR}}$, and get the result, $\boxed{=}$. What do the labels $\boxed{\text{MR}}$, $\boxed{\text{CM}}$, $\boxed{\text{M}+}$, and $\boxed{\text{M}-}$ stand for?

. . . .

$\boxed{\text{MR}}$ means memory recall, i.e., recall from storage.

$\boxed{\text{CM}}$ means clear memory, i.e., empty storage of all numbers except 0.

$\boxed{\text{M}+}$ means add to memory, i.e., place in storage the sum of the last number keyed and the number already in storage.

$\boxed{\text{M}-}$ means subtract from memory, i.e., place in storage the result of subtracting the last number keyed from the number already in storage.

524. Assume that the following sequence is carried out: $\boxed{c}$, $\boxed{CM}$, $\boxed{7}$, $\boxed{\times}$, $\boxed{9}$, $\boxed{=}$, $\boxed{M+}$, $\boxed{4}$, $\boxed{\times}$, $\boxed{2}$, $\boxed{=}$, $\boxed{M-}$, $\boxed{4}$, $\boxed{\div}$, $\boxed{2}$, $\boxed{=}$, $\boxed{M+}$, $\boxed{MR}$. What result do you expect to see on the display?

. . . .

57

$\boxed{c}$ $\boxed{CM}$ *clear both calculator and memory.*

$\boxed{7}$, $\boxed{\times}$, $\boxed{9}$, $\boxed{=}$, $\boxed{M+}$ *places 63 in storage.*

$\boxed{4}$, $\boxed{\times}$, $\boxed{2}$, $\boxed{=}$, $\boxed{M-}$ *subtracts 8 from 63 and leaves 55 in storage.*

$\boxed{4}$, $\boxed{+}$, $\boxed{2}$, $\boxed{=}$, $\boxed{M+}$ *adds 2 to 55 and leaves 57 in storage.*

$\boxed{MR}$ *recalls 57 to the display.*

525. Assume the following sequence has been carried out: $\boxed{c}$, $\boxed{1}$, $\boxed{2}$, $\boxed{\times}$, $\boxed{4}$, $\boxed{\%}$, $\boxed{=}$. What do you expect to see on the display?

. . . .

0.48   *12 X 4% = 12 X 0.04 = 0.48*

526. Assume the following sequence has been carried out: $\boxed{c}$, $\boxed{1}$, $\boxed{2}$, $\boxed{\times}$, $\boxed{4}$, $\boxed{\div}$, $\boxed{100}$, $\boxed{=}$. What do you expect to see on the display?

. . . .

0.48   *12 X 4 = 48   48 ÷ 100 = 0.48*

527. From Frames 525 and 526 we see that to find a percent, one may either press

the % key if the calculator has one, or press two keys, $\boxed{\div}$, $\boxed{100}$. Thus having

a % key saves a little time and effort but is not essential unless one expects to be
doing a great many problems using percents.

Considerations in Choosing a Calculator

528. There are many different types of calculators available.* For daily problems in
nursing, the simplest model is quite sufficient. More complicated models with
keys for trigonometric and exponential functions should be considered if the calculator is to be used for, say, advanced courses in chemistry.

   The simplest model will have keys for the digits 0, 1, 2, ... 9, for the decimal point and equal sign, and for the basic operations, +, −, ×, and ÷. There
will be a key to clear the machine for the next problem; there should also be a
key for clearing the last entry in case of error. All keys should be comfortable
to the touch, not too difficult to press (time-consuming and tiring), or too easy
(causing unintended entries). Sometimes keys are used for more than one purpose; this may also generate errors.

   Algebraic logic is convenient since keys are pressed in the same order as we
write or think the symbols in our mathematical statements. It is also convenient
to have floating point notation. This makes it possible to rely on the machine
for correct positioning of the decimal point, whatever the nature of the problem.
Fixed point notation usually provides answers rounded to two decimal places;
for the simplest problems, this notation is quite satisfactory. Results appearing
on the display should be legible with respect to size and clarity of symbols.

   Pocket calculators are made to run on battery power. A variety of batteries
are found among the different models but instructions for each model give specific information about appropriate selection of batteries. Battery prices have a
wide range; in most cases, the more expensive ones last longest and are recharge-
able. For some calculators, adapters may be purchased to operate the machine
from an AC electrical outlet and to recharge the batteries.

   When shopping for a calculator, what questions would you ask about each
model?

. . . .

*See *Consumer Reports,* Consumers Union, Mt. Vernon, N.Y., 1975, p. 281.

1. What kind of logic does this model use?

2. How easy is it to press the keys?

3. How clear is the display from a number of different angles?

4. How is the calculator powered?

5. If batteries are used, how long are they expected to last?

6. Can the batteries be recharged?

7. What different mathematical operations can be carried out?

8. Does any key have more than one purpose?

9. Does it have floating decimal notation, or is every answer given to two decimal places?

10. Is it a convenient size and weight?

11. How long a guarantee is available?

12. What procedures are necessary for repairs?

13. (Your own personal ideas.)

_____

14. _____

Illustrative Exercises

The following frames contain illustrative problems that can be solved with the aid of a pocket calculator, if you have one. Be sure to study and follow the instructions that come with your calculator. If you do not have a calculator, the problems may be done with paper and pencil of course; they will provide a good review. For more practice with the calculator and further review of theory, use the calculator to do as many problems as possible from the preceding sections of this text.

529. Find the number of pounds in 384 drams. Write your answer in symbols. Then check.

. . . .

lb. iv.   *c, 384 ÷ 8 =, ÷ 12 =*
                                     See Frames 366–375.

530. Find the number of pounds in ℥ lxvi. Then check.

. . . .

lb. vss   *c, 66 ÷ 12 =*

                                     Check: c, 5.5 × 12 =

                                     See Frames 366—375.

---

531. Express 1.4 ml. in the apothecaries' system. Check.

. . . .

𝕞 xxi   *c, 15 × 1.4 =*

                                     *Check: c, 21 × 0.06 = 1.3. The discrep-
                                     ancy occurs because the commonly
                                     used equivalents are not exact.*

                                     See Frames 455—459.

---

532. Find the ratio strength of 125 ml. of silver nitrate solution containing 0.03 Gm.
silver nitrate.

. . . .

1:5000 $0.03 ÷ 125 = \dfrac{2.4}{10,000} = 1:5000$ *approxi-
                                     mately*

                                     See Frames 460—464.

---

533. Check the results in Frame 532 by finding the amount of pure drug in 125 ml.
of a 1:5000 solution.

. . . .

0.03 Gm.   *1 ÷ 5000 × 125 = 0.03*

                                     See Frames 470—479.

---

534. Find the percent strength of 0.8 ml. of atropine sulfate ophthalmic solution containing 4 mg. of pure drug.

. . . .

$\dfrac{1}{2}$% $0.004 ÷ 0.8 = 0.005 = 0.5\%$ *or* $\dfrac{1}{2}$%

                                     See Frames 460—464.

535. Check by finding the amount of pure drug in 0.8 ml. of a 0.5% solution.

. . . .

4 mg.

0.8 × 0.5% = 0.8 × 0.005 = 0.004 Gm. or
4 mg.

See Frames 470–479.

536. In 650 ounces of solution, 1:500, how much boric acid is present? Check.

. . . .

1.3 ounce

650 ÷ 500 = 1.3

Check: 1.3 ÷ 650 = 0.002 = 2:1000 =
1:500

See Frames 470–479.

537. How many milligrams of thiamine are present in 2000 milligrams of a 15% solution of thiamine? Check.

. . . .

300 mg.

2000 × 15% = 300

Check: 300 ÷ 2000 = 0.15 = 15%

See Frames 470–479.

538. You may have on hand boric acid, 1:400, but a patient requires 80 ounces of boric acid, $\frac{1}{500}$. What procedure would you follow?

(Determine the number of ounces (x) of boric acid in 80 ounces of the desired solution, $\frac{1}{500}$. Then find out how many ounces (y) of stock solution, 1:400 must be used. Check.)

. . . .

Use 64 ounces of stock solution and 16 ounces of water to make 80 ounces of the desired solution.

1 ÷ 500 × 80 × 400 = 64

Check: 1 ÷ 400 × 64 ÷ 80 = 0.002 = $\frac{1}{500}$

See Frames 482–491.

539. Nitromersol 1:1000 is to be diluted in order to prepare 180 ml. of nitromersol 1:5000 for use as a disinfectant. How much nitromersol 1:1000 should be used? Check your result.

. . . .

36 ml.

$$\frac{1}{5000} \times 180 \times 1000 = 36 \ ml.$$

Check: $\frac{1}{1000} \times 36 = 0.036,$

$$\frac{0.036}{180} = \frac{2}{10,000} = \frac{1}{5000}$$

See Frames 482–491.

540. Suppose 6 ml. of boric acid, 1:400, were to be prepared with 0.002 Gm. tablets. How many tablets would be needed? Check.

. . . .

$7\frac{1}{2}$

$1 \div 400 \times 6 \div 0.002 = 7.5 \ or \ 7\frac{1}{2}$

$7.5 \times 0.002 \div 6 = 0.0025 = \frac{25}{10,000} = \frac{1}{400}$

See Frames 492–497.

541. How many 2-mg. tablets of reserpine will be needed to make 3.5 cc. of 1:400 solution? Check.

. . . .

4 tablets

$1 \div 400 \times 3.5 \times 1000 \div 2$

Check: $8 \div 3500 = 0.0023 = 1:400$ approximately

See Frames 492–497.

542. How would you prepare 0.4 ml. of a 10% solution of prednisolone acetate using 5 mg. tablets? Check.

. . . .

Dissolve 8 tablets

0.4 × 0.10 × 1000 ÷ 5

Check: 8 × 5 ÷ 1000 ÷ 0.4 = 0.1 = 10%

See Frames 492—497.

---

543. If 3 pints of 1:2000 solution of potassium permanganate were needed to wash out a stomach and 0.2 Gm. scored tablets were on hand, how would you proceed?

. . . .

Dissolve 4 tablets with enough water to make 3 pints of solution.

1 ÷ 2000 × 1500 ÷ 0.2

See Frames 492—497.

---

544. In how much water should a 0.4-Gm. tablet of drug *P* be dissolved in order to have a 0.9% solution? Check.

. . . .

44 ml.

0.4 ÷ 0.009 − 0.4

See Frames 492—497.

Check: 44 + 0.4 = 44.4

0.4 ÷ 44.4 = 0.009 = 0.9%

---

545. Find the number of cc. of solution to measure from a 2.5 cc. vial containing 0.5 Gm. of pure drug if the prescribed dose is 0.3 Gm. Check.

. . . .

1.5 cc.

0.3 ÷ 0.5 × 2.5 = 1.5

Check: 1.5 ÷ 2.5 × 0.5 = 0.3

See Frames 499—503.

---

546. How much atropine would you give a child weighing 28 pounds if orders call for 0.01 mg. per kg.?

. . . .

0.13 mg.

c, 28 ÷ 2.2 × 0.01 = 0.127

See Frames 516—518.

547. A 180 lb. patient is to receive 0.8 mg. of neomycin sulfate per kg. of body weight per day in doses given every 4 hours. How much is this per dose?

. . . .

10.9 mg. $180 \div 2.2 \times 0.8 \div 6$

                                           See Frames 516—518.

548. Suppose the usual adult dose of a drug is 0.4 Gm. Find the doses to be given to the following children: Alice (6 months old), Betty (34 lbs.), Mike (9 years and 2 months old).

. . . .

Alice: 16 mg. $\frac{6}{150} \times 0.4 = 0.016$

Betty: 91 mg. $\frac{34}{150} \times 0.4 = 0.091$

Mike: 171 mg. $\frac{9}{21} \times 0.4 = 0.171$

                                           See Frames 509—515.

APPENDIX

TABLE A
Apothecaries' System of Weights

60 grains = 1 dram
 8 drams = 1 ounce
12 ounces = 1 pound

TABLE B
Apothecaries' System of Fluid Capacity

60 minims   = 1 fluidram
 8 fluidrams   = 1 fluid ounce
16 fluid ounces = 1 pint
 2 pints   = 1 quart
 4 quarts   = 1 gallon

TABLE C
Metric System of Linear Measurement

1000 millimeters = 1 meter
 100 centimeters = 1 meter
  10 meters   = 1 dekameter
 100 meters   = 1 hectometer
1000 meters   = 1 kilometer
                   (approximately 0.6 mile)

TABLE D
Metric System of Weights

1000 micrograms = 1 milligram
1000 milligrams = 1 gram
  10 grams   = 1 dekogram
 100 grams   = 1 hectogram
1000 grams   = 1 kilogram

TABLE E
Metric System of Capacity

1000 milliliters = 1 liter
   10 liters   = 1 dekaliter
  100 liters   = 1 hectoliter
 1000 liters   = 1 kiloliter

TABLE F
Temperature Equivalents

Number of Degrees Fahrenheit (°F)	Number of Degrees Celsius (°C)
32	0
98.6	37
212	100

$$°C = \frac{5}{9} \left(°F - 32°\right)$$

$$°F = 32° + \frac{9}{5} °C$$

TABLE G
Commonly Used Approximate Equivalents

Household	Metric		Apothecaries'	
	Volume	Weight	Volume	Weight
	1 milliliter (ml.) or 1 cubic centimeter (cc.)	1 gram (Gm.)	15 minims	15 grains
1 drop (gtt.)	0.06 ml.	0.06 Gm.	1 minim	1 grain
1 scant teaspoonful (t.)	4 ml.	4 Gm.	1 fluidram	1 dram
2 tablespoonsful (T.)	30 ml.	30 Gm.	1 fluid ounce	1 ounce
1 glassful			8 fluid ounces	
1 pound (avoirdupois not apothecary)	500 ml.		1 pint	
2.2 pounds (avoirdupois, not apothecary)	1 liter (L.)	1 kilogram (kg.)	1 quart	

INDEX